THIS BOOK BELONGS TO

The Library of

....

....

@COPYRIGHT 2024

Thank you for Purchasing my book and taking the time to read it from front to back. I am always grateful when a reader chooses my work and I hope you enjoyed it!

With the vast selection available online, I am touched that you chose to be purchasing my work and take valuable time out of your life to read it. My hope is that you feel you made the right decision.

I very much would like to know what you thought of the book. Please take the time to write an honest and informative review on Amazon.com. Your experience and opinions will be of great benefit to me and those readers looking to make an informed choice.

With much thanks.

Table of Contents

Introduction

Hypertension was often described as a 'silent killer.' While symptoms are commonly absent, persistently elevated blood pressure causes long-term damage to numerous organs and can lead to cardiovascular disease, severe kidney damage, and stroke, and is a significant cause of premature death rates. Hypertension imposes a staggering global burden on the resources of human life quality and the health care system. Hypertension is the primary diagnosis, which is the most common. Even a slight decline shift in the blood pressure distribution in the general public could have a significant impact on cardiovascular risk.

Reducing blood pressure in patients with hypertension of all ages can minimize cardiovascular risk and, in future years, should demonstrate to be of significant economic benefit. Numerous hypertension communities worldwide have endorsed intensive blood pressure control and the significance of pharmacological intervention in specific high-risk individuals with hypertension.

In addition to providing more effective, well-tolerated blood pressure control, the primary objective of antihypertensive therapy should be to reduce cardiovascular disease and discourage premature death. Studies have shown convincingly that antihypertensive operatives can lower stroke risks. Even minor declines in blood pressure bring meaningful benefits. High blood pressure can not only be prevented with medication and drugs. Instead, it is more beneficial to control high blood pressure with diet and a significant change in lifestyle naturally.

Dietary changes have been widely viewed as a lifestyle change strategy with enormous potential to prevent hypertension at a cost that is often lower than current pharmacological interventions. Such practical historical approaches are reflected in dietary recommendations advocating weight loss, reduced dietary sodium intake, and restraint in alcohol consumption, and more recently revised to reflect the lowering effect of potassium supplementation on blood pressure and a dietary eating pattern. This book reviews the consistency of the results of blood pressure concerning proven dietary interventions and several new dietary targets.

A variety of dietary changes are beneficial in treating hypertension, including a reduction in sodium intake, alcohol moderation, weight loss in overweight or obese, and a diet rich in fruits, vegetables, legumes, and low-fat dairy products and low in snacks, sweets, meat, and saturated fat. Individual dietary factors may also reduce blood pressure (BP).

Also, consideration should be given to non-dietary lifestyle modification modalities, including termination of smoking and establishment of an aerobic exercise regime. Most no pharmacological therapy studies assessed only one factor to prove its effectiveness (e.g., weight reduction without sodium restriction). However, in making a recommendation to the individual patient, the clinician will try to alter all of the variables that may contribute to the BP elevation, although it is uncertain whether the effects of various modifications are additive.

Lifestyle changes in those with elevated BP or stage 1 hypertension may adequately control the BP. However, drug therapies should first be used among those with either high BP or additional risk (e.g., diabetes or chronic kidney disease) to control the BP more quickly and effectively; Once the BP is well regulated, changes in lifestyle should be highly recommended.

If these lifestyles have been achieved successfully, it may be possible to reduce the number of medications.

Chapter 1: High Blood Pressure or Hypertension

Normal blood pressure has vital importance to life. Not any nutrients or oxygen would be distributed to the organs and tissues through our arteries without the friction that causes our blood to circulate across the circulatory system. Blood pressure is important because the higher your blood pressure is, the higher your risk of health problems in the future. Blood pressure can get dangerously high, though, and it can also get too low.

We discuss in this chapter about what blood pressure is and how it is calculated. What the measures mean for our health, disorders of blood pressure, causes, and symptoms of blood pressure, and medication for treating high blood pressure.

1.1 What Is Blood Pressure and How It Is Measured

Blood pressure is a force that blood exerts in the arteries as it circulates. It is classified into systolic pressures (a contraction of the heart) and diastolic pressures (filling of the heart).

In simple words, blood pressure is the force that pushes blood across the circulatory system.

It is an important force because, without blood pressure, oxygen, and nutrients cannot be move through our circulatory system to nurture organs and tissues.

Blood pressure is also important as it offers protection for white blood cells, antibodies, and hormones, such as insulin.

Just as essential as supplying nutrients and oxygen, the fresh blood that is supplied is capable of storing metabolic, toxic waste items such as the carbon dioxide that we exhale with every intake and the contaminants that we flush from our liver and kidneys.

Blood itself has several other characteristics, including its temperature. It also holds one of our protections against harm to the tissue, the clotting platelets, which prevent blood loss after injury.

But what specifically does blood allow our arteries to create pressure? Part of the explanation is straightforward by squeezing blood out when its contract with every pulse, the heart produces blood pressure. However, blood pressure cannot be specifically created by the heart beating.

High Blood Pressure

High blood pressure is a widely common condition in which the long-term force of the blood opposing your artery walls is high enough that it may eventually cause health problems. Blood pressure is determined both by two things.

The amount of blood your heart pumps as well as the amount of resistance to blood flow in your arteries. The rule is that the more blood your heart pumps and the narrower your arteries, the higher your blood pressure.

Function

Our circulation is identical to a highly sophisticated plumbing process blood has 'flow' and arteries are 'pipes.' A simple law of physics ultimately leads to our blood flow, and this law often relates to a garden hose pump. Blood flows throughout our bodies, leading to a pressure difference. Our blood pressure is highest from our heart at the beginning of its journey-when it enters the aorta-and it is weakest at the end of its journey across progressively smaller artery branches. The difference in pressure is what allows blood to flow across our bodies.

Arteries have a similar effect on blood pressure to the physical properties of a garden hose pipe, which influences water pressure. Tightening the pipe at the level of constriction increases the pressure.

For starters, without the elasticity of the artery walls, blood pressure will drop faster as it's drained from the heart.

While the heart produces the maximum pressure, it is just as important to maintain the properties of the arteries and to enable blood to flow through the whole body.

Measurement

The tool which is used to assess blood pressure is a sphygmomanometer, which consists of a rubber armband, the manual or electronic pump inflated belt.

Once the cuff is fully filled to interrupt the pulse, a reading is taken, whether electronically or on an analog dial.

The reading is measured by the pressure required to move mercury across a tube toward gravity. This is the reason the metric millimeters of mercury abbreviated to mm Hg is used to calculate pressure.

Measuring blood pressure seems to be the only way to determine if you have hypertension. High blood pressure typically has no indicators or effects, and many people don't know they have it.

How Do Health Care Professionals Measure Blood Pressure?

First, a medical practitioner puts an inflatable band around your arm. Afterward, the medical practitioner pumps up the cuff, which tightens softly on the arm. The cuff has a measuring gauge on it that measures your blood pressure.

By listening to your heartbeat with a stethoscope and monitoring the gauge, the medical practitioner will gradually release air out from the cuff. That is a painless and quick operation. The medical practitioner will not have to use a stethoscope when using an electronic or automated blood pressure cuff.

To assess the pressure into your arteries, the instrument uses a weighing unit called mercury millimeters (mmHg).

When you have high blood pressure, explore steps to take to manage your blood pressure and lower heart disease risk and stroke with your healthcare team.

How Can Blood Pressure Be Measure At Home?

Your health care provider regarding checking the blood pressure at home on a regular basis, often known as self-measured blood pressure control (SMBP).

SMBP means you use a private blood pressure measuring device regularly away from your doctor's office or hospital, usually at home. Such blood pressure monitoring devices are user-friendly and discreet. A member of the health care team can demonstrate to you how to use one in case you need help.

Evidence indicates that individuals with high blood pressure are much more likely to reduce their blood pressure when using SMBP in addition to assistance from their healthcare team than when using SMBP without any healthcare team.

How Often Should Blood Pressure Be Measured?

Talk to your doctor or to your health care provider about how often your blood pressure should be checked, or when it should be calculated by yourself. People with high blood pressure will continue to more regularly check their blood pressure than persons who don't have high blood pressure.

What Should You Do If Your Numbers Are High?

If your blood pressure numbers make you worried then talk to your healthcare team. They can help you formulate a plan for managing high blood pressure. You can also take steps every day just to help keep your blood pressure within a healthy range, and it does not matter how old you are.

Facts about High Blood Pressure or Hypertension

You might get hurt by what you don't actually understand regarding high blood pressure. High blood pressure impacts one in three persons, yet it is not recognized by many people with the disease.

Unmonitored high blood pressure increases the risk of heart disease and stroke and may also lead to death causes. High blood pressure is thankfully preventable and treatable. Have your blood pressure regularly tested to lower your risk and take action to manage your blood pressure if it becomes too high.

High Blood Pressure Linked To Dementia

Researches show that high blood pressure is associated with a higher risk of dementia, a collapse of cognitive function. Timing does seem to matter some evidence indicates that uncontrolled high blood pressure all through midlife (age 45 to 65) leads to a higher risk of dementia later in life.

Young People Also Have High Blood Pressure

High blood pressure not only occurs in older adults. About one in three people and almost one in four women between the ages of 35 and 44 have high blood pressure. High blood pressure is the main cause of stroke. Experts believe that the increased risk of stroke among young adults results directly from rising obesity rates, high blood pressure, and diabetes conditions that can be prevented and treated.

Young people should be getting their blood pressure checked regularly.

Most people who have high blood pressure don't even realize that they have. The only way to know that is to regularly check your blood pressure.

High Blood Pressure Usually Doesn't Show Any Symptoms

Often, high blood pressure is considered the "silent killer." Many individuals with high blood pressure have no signs, like sweating or headaches. As many individuals feel fine, they don't consider their blood pressure needs to be checked. Even if you're feeling fine, your health could be at risk. Consult your doctor about the risk of developing high blood pressure.

Many Peoples Who Have High Blood Pressure Don't Know It

Many peoples with high blood pressure aren't even aware of it and don't get medical attention to regulate their blood pressure. Most patients with high blood pressure have healthcare insurance and at least twice a year see a health care provider, but the disease stays undiagnosed, unnoticed from the patients and doctors. CDC works with operators to find high blood pressure patients who are "near in sight." Consult the health care provider what does your blood pressure results mean or if they are too high. If you are dealing with high blood pressure, stick to your course of treatment, and seek the provider's recommendations.

Women and Minorities Especially Face Unique Risks When It Comes To High Blood Pressure

Females who become pregnant with high blood pressure are more likely to experience risks during childbirth as compared to those who have normal blood pressure. High blood pressure may destroy the kidneys of a mother and other organs and may cause low birth weight and premature delivery. Certain kinds of birth control can also increase the risk of high blood pressure for a woman. Women who have high blood pressure and wish to become pregnant must consult with their health care advisor before becoming pregnant to reduce their blood pressure.

African American males and females exhibit higher blood pressure rates than any other culture or race. Such people are more likely to be admitted to hospital with high blood pressure. Many experts believe that this has to do with higher obesity rates, diabetes, and stroke among a certain group. Changes in lifestyle such as the salt reduction in your diet, greater physical activity, and stress reduction, may significantly lower blood pressure.

Systolic and Diastolic Pressure

When the heart pumps blood through your lungs, it moves the blood under a pressure head up. Physicians calculate your blood pressure as a means to determine the impact that flowing blood exerts on the lining of your arteries.

Although the heartbeats through the lungs is not constant (as with a fire hose), but pulsatile, and the blood flow and the intensity that it exerts fluctuates from moment to time.

For this purpose, a person's blood pressure level is reported as two separate figures the systolic blood pressure and the diastolic blood pressure. These two numbers represent various aspects of the energy the blood is exerting as it flows through your arteries.

The systolic and diastolic pressures are both significant. If the levels are too high, there may be hypertension. Unless the blood pressure levels are too low, the blood flow to vital organs like the brain may not be enough.

What Is Systolic Blood Pressure?

The pressure placed by blood flow into your arteries is not continuous but is dynamic and is a constant reflection of what the heart is doing at a given time.

When the heart beats vigorously, (an event called "systole"), blood is pumped out in the arteries. This complex blood ejection into the arteries is causing pressure to increase inside the arteries. The highest blood pressure reached through active contracting of the heart is considered the systolic blood pressure.

A "standard" systolic blood pressure when a person sitting comfortably is at or below 120 mmHg.

High Systolic Blood Pressure

When a person is doing exercise during times of mental stress or at any other moment when the heart is induced to pump more strongly than in rest, the frequency of heart contraction rises, and the systolic pressure increases. The rise of systolic blood pressure that happens during these cardiac stress situations is completely normal. That explains why measuring blood pressure during quiet rest periods before assessing hypertension is so important.

Low Systolic Blood Pressure

If the systolic blood pressure is less than usual, the occurrence of systolic hypotension is recorded. If systolic hypotension is too serious, then lightheadedness, dizziness, syncope, or organ failure will occur. Systolic hypotension can occur when the blood volume becomes too weak (such as with severe dehydration or a large bleeding episode) when the heart muscle becomes too sluggish to expel the blood usually (a condition known as cardiomyopathy) or when the blood vessels become too dilated (such as in vasovagal syncope). One common condition resulting in systolic hypotension is orthostatic hypotension.

What Is Diastolic Blood Pressure?

Diastolic blood pressure is actually the pressure that the blood exerts during heartbeats inside the arteries, that is when the heart does not actively pump blood into the arteries. After the heartbeats, the cardiac ventricles relax slightly in anticipation of the next contraction so they can be refilled from the blood. This time period of ventricular relaxation is called "diastole," and the blood pressure is called diastolic blood pressure during diastole.

Normal, High, and Low Diastolic Blood Pressure

During quiet rest, a "normal" diastolic blood pressure is 80 mmHg or less. In hypertension, the diastolic blood pressure is sometimes increased during quiet rest.

Diastolic hypotension (when the blood pressure becomes low) can be seen with dehydration or incidents of diarrhea or if the arteries are abnormally dilated.

The Importance of Measuring Blood Pressure During Quiet Rest

Blood pressure is pretty dynamic. Your blood pressure level relies on your cardiac rate and elasticity of the arteries. As we have seen, as the heart cycles among systole and diastole, the blood pressure is consciously shifting from minute to minute.

Additionally, the systolic and diastolic blood pressure can substantially change from moment to moment, depending on your state of activity, stress, hydration status, and several other factors.

What this indicates is that it is important to monitor as many "external" factors as possible in an attempt to detect hypertension appropriately. The standard prescribed by clinicians needs the blood pressure to be measured in a relaxed, warm environment after you've been comfortably sitting for at least five minutes. Monitoring blood pressure like this method is difficult in today's modern, rendering the accurate evaluation of hypertension far more of a problem than it should be. That is why most specialists today advise recording blood pressure through an extended time period, with outpatient monitoring, before having the hypertension diagnosis.

Understanding Blood Pressure Readings

Everyone needs healthy blood pressure. Still, what does that mean exactly?

If the doctor takes your blood pressure, it is represented as a two-number scale, with one digit at the top (systolic) and one at the bottom (diastolic) as a fraction. E.g., 120/80 mm Hg. The numerator represents the amount of strain in your bloodstream during the heart muscle contractions, which is regarded as systolic pressure. The denominator corresponds to your blood pressure when the muscle of your heart is between beats. That is regarded as diastolic pressure. Both numbers are important for assessing heart health status. Numbers above the ideal range show the heart works really hard to pump blood to your whole body.

Normal Reading of Blood Pressure

Blood pressure needs to tell a top number (systolic pressure) between 90 and less than 120 and a bottom number (diastolic pressure) between 60 and less than 80 for normal reading. When both the systolic and diastolic levels are in these percentages, blood pressure is assumed to be within the normal range.

Blood pressure levels are measured in mercury millimeters. This term shall be abbreviated as mm Hg. A blood pressure which is below 120/80 mm Hg and which is above 90/60 mm Hg would be common readings in an adult.

If you are in the normal range, there is no need for medical intervention. You should maintain a healthy diet and a healthy weight to better prevent the development of hypertension. Daily working out and eating well can also benefit. When hypertension exists in your family, you may have to be even more aware of your lifestyles.

Stages of Hypertension

Following are some stages of hypertension to consider:

Elevated Blood Pressure

Numbers above 120/80 mm Hg are a red flag you need to adopt heart-healthy activities. If your systolic pressure varies from 120 to 129 mm Hg and your diastolic pressure is less than 80 mm Hg, that implies you have increased blood pressure. Although these figures are not considered high blood pressure, technically, you have stepped out of the normal range. Elevated blood pressure is likely to turn into real high blood pressure, placing you at a higher risk of heart disease and stroke.

There is no need for treatment for elevated blood pressure. But this is when you need to adopt healthier lifestyle choices. A nutritious diet and regular exercise will help lower the blood pressure to a normal range and prevent the development of increased blood pressure into full-fledged hypertension.

Hypertension: Stage 1

If your systolic blood pressure exceeds between 130 and 139 mm, Hg or diastolic blood pressure hits between 80 and 89 mm Hg. You will usually be identified with high blood pressure. This is called hypertension stage 1.

However, you may not have very high blood pressure if you only get one reading at this extreme. What decides the hypertension status at any point is the average rate of the numbers over a time period.

Your doctor can help you calculate your blood pressure and monitor it to check if it's too high. If your blood pressure does not improve after one month of following a healthy lifestyle, you may need to start taking drugs, especially if you're already at higher risk for heart disease. If you are at a lower risk, your doctor may also want to follow-up after you have developed more healthy habits within three to six months.

If you are 65 or older and often healthy, the doctor would possibly prescribe improvements in care and diet if your systolic blood pressure reaches 130 mm Hg. The diagnosis should be provided on a case-by-case basis with people 65 and over who have major health problems.

Treatment of high blood pressure in elderly people seems to reduce memory and dementia problems.

Hypertension: Stage 2

Stage 2 suggests another more serious condition with high blood pressure. If your reading of the blood pressure indicates a top number of 140 or even more, or a low number of 90 or more, hypertension is called level 2.

Your doctor will prescribe one or more drugs at this point to keep your blood pressure in order. But for managing hypertension, you should not depend solely on medicines. In stage 2, the lifestyle habits are often just as critical as in the other phases.

Such drugs that can support a healthy lifestyle include:

- ACE antagonists that prevent blood vessel contracting substances
- Alpha-blockers used to loosen arteries
- Beta-blockers to decrease heart rate and remove substances that widen blood vessels
- Calcium channel blockers to relieve blood vessels and decrease heart function
- Diuretics to reduce the amount of fluid in your body

Danger Zone

Measurement of blood pressure above 180/120 mm Hg shows a significant health problem. Such elevated levels are referred to as a "hypertensive problem." Blood pressure above this range demands immediate care even though no associated signs occur.

When you have blood pressure above this range, you should receive medical care which could follow signs like:

- Chest In Pain
- Visual Changes
- Symptoms of Stroke
- Blood In Your Urine
- Shortness of Breath
- Headache
- Dizziness

Sometimes a high reading of blood pressure can occur momentarily, and then the numbers return to regular. If your blood pressure measures at this stage, your physician should typically take a second reading within a few minutes. A second high reading means that you will require care either as early as possible or urgently, based on whether you have all of the above-described symptoms or not.

Preventive Measures

If you have good levels, protective steps will be taken to maintain the blood pressure within limits. This will help you reduce the chances of cholesterol, heart failure, and stroke.

Prevention is much more important as you start aging. Systolic pressure begins to crawl up until you're past 50, so that's even more significant trusted source to estimate coronary heart attack incidence and other conditions. Other health problems may also play a part, such as diabetes and kidney failure. Speak to the doctor on how physical health should be controlled to better avoid the development of hypertension.

Blood Pressure that's Too Low

The low blood pressure is referred to as hypotension. For adults, a level of 90/60 mm Hg or less of blood pressure is also called hypotension. It can be risky as the very low blood pressure will not provide sufficiently oxygenated blood to the body and heart.

Other possible triggers of hypotension may include:

- Heart Problems
- **Dehydration**
- **Pregnancy**
- Blood Loss
- Severe Infection (Septicemia)
- **Anaphylaxis**
- **Malnutrition**
- Endocrine Problems
- Certain Medications

Hypotension usually coincides with light-headedness or dizziness. Speak to the doctor regarding the existence of your low blood pressure and what you should do to increase your blood pressure.

Blood Pressure Chart

In order to control your blood pressure, you need to learn which figures of blood pressure are good, and which ones trigger the alarm. Following are levels of blood pressure used to treat adult's hypotension and hypertension.

Hypotension usually refers more to signs and particular conditions than to absolute figures.

Hypotension figures act as a reference, while hypertension statistics are more precise.

Blood Pressure Category	Systolic(Top Number)	Diastolic(Bottom Number)
Hypotension	90 or below	60 or Below
Normal	91 to 119	61 To 79
Elevated	Between 120 and 129	And Below 80
Stage 1 hypertension	Between 130 and 139	or Between 80 And 89
Stage 2 hypertension	140 or higher	or 90 or Higher
Hypertensive crisis	Higher than 180	Higher Than120

Note that just one of them has to be so high to place you in a hypertensive group while looking at certain figures. If your blood pressure is 119/81, for example, you should be known to have hypertension in stage 1.

Blood Pressure Levels for Children

Blood pressure levels for children vary from those for adults. Blood pressure levels for children are calculated by multiple variables, such as:

- Age
- Gender
- Height

When you are worried about their blood pressure, speak to your child's pediatrician. The pediatrician will talk to you through the charts to help you recognize blood pressure from your kids.

How to Take a Reading

There are a few options to get your blood pressure tested. Your doctor can test your blood pressure in their clinic, for example. Most hospitals now provide blood pressure control stations free of charge. Professional blood pressure monitoring will even try things out at home. This may be bought from the pharmacy and medical supplies shops.

Use an automated home blood pressure cuff that monitors blood pressure on the upper arm. Blood pressure sensors for the hand or finger are still available but might not be as accurate.

1.2 Disorders of Blood Pressure (Fluctuating BP)

Some doctor's clinic visits may include a test of blood pressure. This is because your blood pressure will say a lot about your health to the doctor. A number that is relatively low or somewhat high can be a symbol of future issues. Increases in blood pressure during appointments may also be a sign of health conditions.

Your blood pressure is a measurement of the intensity through the circulatory system through which blood flows. Obviously, blood pressure varies several times a day. Many improvements are gradual and natural. You do not experience noticeable signs or effects when these fluctuations arise in the blood pressure. Those can be short and transient variations. Know more concerning levels in blood pressure.

But, if you find that the levels of high pressure are very high or that the levels of low pressure are really low, you might want to speak to the doctor. Once such improvements are detected, it is important that you note them in a log. Write down the figures, the activities, and also how long it took to get back to work with the figure. Such knowledge will help you or your doctor to identify a problem.

Causes of Fluctuating Blood Pressure

Many factors may cause fluctuating blood pressure.

Stress

Emotional tension and anxiety may raise blood pressure for a temporary duration. With time, constant tension will affect the cardiovascular system, which may contribute to lifelong issues with blood pressure.

White-Coat Syndrome

White-coat syndrome happens when anxiety or discomfort triggers a sudden increase in blood pressure following a doctor's visit. You can consider your reading routine at home. A diagnosis with lower blood pressure does not indicate that you have hypertension (severe blood pressure). Those with white-coat hypertension, though, are more prone to have high blood pressure.

Medication

All over-the-counter medicines and prescribed drugs will influence blood pressure. Many medical drugs, such as diuretics and blood pressure medication, are intended to reduce blood pressure. Others may raise blood pressure, such as cold and allergy drugs.

Activity

Exercising, chatting, laughing, and even sex may induce changes in blood pressure.

Food and Drink

What you drink or eat, it may have an effect on reading your blood pressure. Products rich in tyrosine (a compound common in aged products) can raise blood pressure. This involves foods which include:

- Fermented
- Pickled
- Brined
- Cured
- Drinks with Caffeine Can Boost Blood Pressure Numbers Temporarily

Adrenal Issues

The adrenal system is responsible for the production of hormones. Adrenal exhaustion occurs when the output of hormones is weak. This can result in blood pressure falling. An overactive adrenal system may cause the blood pressure and hypertension to unexpectedly spikes.

Pheochromocytoma

This unusual tumor arises in the adrenal glands, which inhibits the development of hormones. With typical intervals in between, it may trigger abrupt spikes of abnormal blood pressure readings.

Risk Factors of Fluctuation of Blood Pressure

Such factors can put you at greater risk of fluctuating blood pressure:

- High levels of stress
- Anxiety
- Taking blood pressure pills that aren't effective or don't last until your next dose
- Tobacco use
- Excessive alcohol consumption
- Night-shift work

In fact, other factors may raise the likelihood of having fluctuating blood pressure. Including:

- Diabetes
- Pregnancy
- Dehydration
- Cardiovascular disease
- Poorly controlled or uncontrolled high blood pressure
- Obstructive sleep apnea
- kidney disease
- Thyroid problems
- Nervous system problems

Complications of Fluctuating Blood Pressure

Fluctuating blood pressure levels aren't necessarily an indicator of a greater health concern, although it may be a warning sign of potential issues for certain patients. Including:

Hypertension

Hypertension may not progress quickly. It's always a slow upward change, so odd readings may be the first indication of a problem. Always screen for symptoms of persistent hypertension to monitor the blood pressure.

Heart Disease

For one report, patients with changes in blood pressure during hospital visits were more prone to experience heart disease and stroke than those who had regular rates of blood pressure.

Dementia

One research showed that individuals with fluctuations of blood pressure were twice as likely as individuals without fluctuation to experience this mental deterioration.

Who Is Most Likely To Develop High Blood Pressure?

- Smokers
- People with a family history of having high blood pressure
- Pregnant women
- Women who take birth control pills
- Those over the age of 35
- People who are overweight or obese
- Inactive people
- Those who drink too much alcohol
- Those who eat too many fatty foods or foods with too much salt consumption
- People having sleep apnea

1.3 Causes of High Blood Pressure

High blood pressure is, however, a major cause of death, provided that cardiac disease and stroke are main victims.

For this reason, it is critical that you know about this silent killer as much as you can. One way to remain healthy from high blood pressure problems is to perform routine blood pressure checks. This means you will make sure you have a track of it. But what makes blood pressure high? This is a difficult problem.

Following are some of the common causes of hypertension:

Advanced Age

Though age is not solely a reason for high blood pressure, risks of hypertension rise with age. Around 80 percent of individuals aged 65 and over are reported to have hypertension. Generally, individuals above the age of 55 have a greater chance of having high blood pressure.

It can be due to changes that develop over time, such as decreased blood vessel capacity, decreased salt sensitivity, hormonal shifts, and decreased heart performance. That ensures that although anyone can routinely have their blood pressure checked, elderly adults can take it even more seriously.

Obesity

In comparison to certain health issues, if you are overweight or obese, you are at a greater risk of having high blood pressure. The same goes for individuals with heavy fat reserves in their abdomen, thighs, and buttocks. About 70 percent of people are projected to be overweight. Excess weight is typically attributed to inadequate nutrition, unhealthy lifestyle, and lack of exercise. Obesity is considered one of the factors for the increase in high blood pressure in recent decades.

In the case that your body frame has a higher body mass index than average, you will perform routine blood pressure tests. You should also take measures to reduce the weight by having a healthy diet, physical exercise, and avoidance of stress.

Stress

The stress allows the blood pressure to increase temporarily. This is not the same as hypertension. Even as blood pressure increases regularly, it may impact the strength of the blood vessels and eventually contribute to high blood pressure development. Yet experiments do not support this. But persistent stress may contribute to hormonal imbalances. This may even lead you to engage in activities such as drug addiction, overeating, or difficulty sleeping. It is understood that certain factors trigger high blood pressure. Regardless of how high blood pressure contributes to stress, you can do everything you can to prevent adverse situations. Activities such as meditation, yoga, and aerobic activity may also reduce tension.

Alcohol Consumption

Numerous studies have shown that regular alcohol intake can contribute to hypertension. This can involve consuming more than three servings daily. Although drinking one or two drinks a day can have no negative health consequences, having more than three in seating allows the blood pressure to increase instantly. If this occurs periodically, the long-term blood pressure that can eventually contribute to hypertension can stay elevated.

When you have high blood pressure, reduce or stop your alcohol consumption may help in improvements. It is important to remember that women have a greater sensitivity to drug usage than males. So women should restrict their alcohol consumption to one drink a day and men should restrict their alcohol intake to two.

Sedentary Lifestyle

Whether you're stuck at work or at home for long hours, you're a target for high blood pressure. That is because only the calories the body requires for maintenance are burned. This is different from an individual whose job involves physical exertion. A sedentary lifestyle can often lead the body to keep fluid in the lower sections, such as knees, feet, and thighs. Retention of fluid may often contribute to increased blood pressure.

If your job requires you a lot of sitting, build a pattern of taking breaks for walking around during the day. You may also opt to go walking when going to or from the job. Alternatively, participate in a gym to work out at least one hour to a half every week.

Smoking

A further leading indicator of high blood pressure is tobacco smoke. Cigarette smoke includes various chemicals that have harmful health consequences. Many of these compounds allow atherosclerosis to grow, which includes the narrowing of the blood vessels. This ensures the heart needs to perform extra work to pump blood into the narrowed blood vessels. The spike in blood pressure is what is known as hypertension.

If you are a tobacco smoker, it's best to stop regardless of whether you have hypertension or not. This will help to reduce your blood pressure or decrease the chance of having it. Aside from many safety problems, smoking is often believed to cause cancer.

Diet

Whatever you consume has a huge effect on your general health. Eating diets rich in cholesterol, sugar, and salt. For example, it will contribute to high blood pressure rising. This is understood that salt, sugar, and high carbohydrate diets raise body weight, as well as adipose fat in the chest, thighs, and hips. High blood pressure is believed to induce extra body weight and fat deposits.

When you have high blood pressure, try consuming a balanced diet that is low in calories, sugar, and salt and rich in fruits and vegetables. You can always take sufficient fluids to keep you hydrated and help lower your consumption of calories. Therefore, advised that everyone should consume a balanced diet to reduce the incidence of hypertension.

Excess Salt Intake

Although table salt helps enhance the flavor of food, it may cause high blood pressure if consumed in significant doses. Reports often show certain individuals are more prone to salt than others are. This suggests some individuals are more prone to have high blood pressure than the others, even though they take salt in equal quantities. If you have increased blood pressure, so try lowering the consumption of sodium.

Reducing the consumption of salt will also significantly reduce the chance of developing hypertension. This should be remembered that much of the refined products produce large quantities of salt. And if you intend to minimize the salt consumption, skip fried products and scan the labeling closely if you choose to consume them.

Some Medications

Daily intake of some medicines may induce hypertension. There is a long-range of medications that may induce hypertension. These contain anti-inflammatory anti-steroidal medications, antibiotics, some birth control pills, and other decongestants. Some of such drugs contribute to high blood pressure by inducing fluid accumulation in the body. Some can trigger blood vessels to widen.

This is best to stop taking needless drugs and to take all medicines as instructed by the doctor. Always think for potential adverse effects and scan the packaging if you receive a prescription. Do keep the doctor aware of any drugs you are taking to eliminate harmful reactions.

Family History

If your family member has, or ever had hypertension, you're at a greater risk of developing it. Several reports have shown that hypertension tends to be occurring through families. Observations have also been produced that citizens of African descent are at greater risk of developing hypertension from those of European, Hispanic, or Asian descent.

These results do not indicate whether you belong to a family or regression with a higher risk for the problem; you would probably get high blood pressure. Knowing you're going to get high blood pressure, however, will encourage you to live a healthy lifestyle. This will greatly be raising the chances of developing the disease. Do note that to maintain things under the balance, and you need to perform daily blood pressure tests and figure out whether you have one.

1.4 Symptoms of High Blood Pressure

High blood pressure is a disorder in which blood pressure increases and persists steadily above 120/80 mm Hg. High blood pressure is commonly known as hypertension (the product of the internal arterial walls being stiffened or hardened). When blood passes into the arteries, this induces excessive resistance. The consequence is that the heart needs to function particularly hard to pump oxygen through the various areas of the body.

This remains unknown what is the real source of hypertension. Although, this typically impacts those with families with a background of increased blood pressure, those who are 50 years of age or older, overweight or obese, those who live sedentary lives, and those who eat too much alcohol or salt. What signs of high blood pressure will you look out for? Since hypertension has no clear effects, in the event of the following signs, you may need to go through blood pressure checks.

Nosebleeds

Nosebleeds, also identified as epistaxis, is one of elevated blood pressure signs common to everyone. It is observed among a small percentage of patients with undiagnosed increased blood pressure as they seek to care for nosebleeds. Research showed that 17 percent of patients admitted at the hospital for accidents of high blood pressure suffered from repeated nosebleeds.

High blood pressure will trigger nosebleeds if any of the tiny blood capillaries inside the nose break down from the pressure. It will allow blood to flow to the capillaries. When you have frequent nosebleeds, the blood pressure is possibly heavy. You have to go for a blood pressure check for this purpose.

Blurred Vision

If high blood pressure continues on unnoticed and untreated, blurry vision will results. It happens because the intense pressure will harden or burst tiny capillaries in the brain. The same may happen with the blood vessels which supply the retina with blood. It interferes with blood flow to other areas of the body.

Consequently, the body, particularly the optic nerve and the retina, in particular, do not obtain enough blood to supply them with both the oxygen and nutrients they need to function properly. If this continues without care for a prolonged period of time, it may induce vision impairment.

Headache

Hypertension is also responsible for headaches. For this cause, several people, like physicians, equate hypertension with other forms of headaches. A study of people with migraine disorders showed that there was high blood pressure among 21 percent of the people. It indicates that while not all with headaches would have hypertension, a significant sign of high blood pressure may be the existence of a headache.

Hypertension symptoms are more likely to develop if there is no explanation of the disorder or whether it is not managed. When you get frequent headaches, you'll definitely need to have hypertension checked. When the test is positive, the doctor can place you on medicine to decrease the blood pressure, which would also decrease the headache frequency and intensity.

Breathlessness

Breathlessness is a sign of hypertensive pulmonary pressure. It is high blood pressure, which influences the pulmonary arteries within the lungs. These arteries will become dense and rigid, which enhances blood resistance passing into them. The resistance contributes to blood pressure elevation.

Pulmonary blood pressure indicates that blood does not pump as freely through the bloodstream as it can, resulting in a loss of sufficient oxygen or nutrients. As the body wants more oxygen and nutrients than the lungs can provide, it is important for the lungs to function harder, which causes breathlessness. Certain pulmonary hypertensive signs cause dizziness, tiredness, and chest pressure.

Fatigue

While there are several factors that may induce exhaustion, high blood pressure can also be a symptom. Blood is the vehicle that supplies all the organs and tissues in the body with oxygen and nutrients. Those are the raw materials that provide the energy that the organs and tissues need to carry out their important functions.

In high blood pressure situations, blood flow is inhibited in such a manner that certain muscles and tissues are deprived of sufficient nutrients and oxygen. Consequently, energy is not generated which is required for the operation of certain body parts, which induces fatigue. In this condition, you may not be able to carry out your everyday tasks effectively. You need to get your blood pressure tested if you are feeling constant exhaustion.

Confusion

Confusion is a sign of high blood pressure strongly linked to fatigue. Like in all body organs and tissues, if the brain does not obtain sufficient levels of oxygen and nutrients, its tasks cannot be done as well as they can. It may contribute to intellectual fatigue and an unwillingness to care for certain visual sensations or interpret them. When you find you are suffering from periods of confusion, blood pressure monitoring is recommended.

Chest Pain

If you have persistent chest pain or discomfort, the blood pressure is possibly heavy. Chest pressure may be followed by respiratory problems and an erratic pulse. That is because the heart will work extremely hard to push blood into arteries that are less flexible.

Heart discomfort or distress is most likely to arise if either the pulmonary arteries that bring blood to the lungs are damaged, or the coronary artery that delivers blood to the heart muscles. In the event of pulmonary blood pressure, the heart will function extremely hard to push blood into the lungs, and in the situation of coronary artery disease, which is a loss of enough oxygen and nutrients can stretch the heart.

Low Libido

High blood pressure will result in low libido and sexual dysfunction. It is most likely to happen in men but it may happen in women as well. Since excessive high blood pressure may destroy the blood vessels, including the vessels that support the penis, the effect could be insufficient blood flow. Sexual impairment exists because it's impossible to obtain or sustain an erection without enough blood circulating through the penis.

Damaged blood vessels in women can indicate that the vagina is not receiving enough blood. It adds to dryness, decreased sexual desire, and trouble having an orgasm. When you experience a drop in sexual libido, you will get your blood pressure tested. Further tests can also be done to find out any health concerns.

Heart Palpitations

A heart palpitation is the sensation of a beat absent from the heart. This will sometimes happen for various reasons. However, it can be a sign of high blood pressure, as heart palpitations arise frequently. Another indication the blood pressure can be extremely high is a pounding pulse. During palpitations, you can experience anxiety, too.

High blood pressure means the heart may have to pump even faster than usual, which will cause it to tire. In fact, high blood pressure may also impact the heart-supplying blood vessels. During this situation, the heart cannot obtain sufficient oxygen and glucose to provide the energy it takes for proper functioning. For these causes, in case you have repeated heart palpitations or rapid heartbeats, you can see a specialist.

Swelling in the Ankles

Swelling in the lower sections of the body, particularly the legs, ankles, and feet, may be a symptom of high blood pressure. The swelling, often called edema, happens when the heart is exhausted and thus cannot do all the activity of pumping. It allows the body to accumulate blood, which absorbs and induces edema inside tissues. For certain instances, edema is an indication that the problem with blood pressure has long been present. This could mean the kidneys already malfunction. The heart can still be seriously impaired and can collapse. Avoid waiting for the edema to leave for these purposes. In contrast, head to a treatment facility to get checked for high blood pressure as well as other complications.

1.5 Medication for Treating High Blood Pressure

Monitoring your blood pressure at home is an effective way to test if a blood pressure medication is successful, to verify that you have high blood pressure, or to monitor rising high blood pressure.

Home blood pressure monitors are common and inexpensive, so you don't need a prescription to purchase one. Home blood pressure control isn't a replacement for the doctor's appointments, so home blood pressure control can have some drawbacks.

Be sure an approved tool is used, and test whether the cuff works. Bring the machine to the doctor's office for an annual test of its accuracy. Speak to your doctor before beginning a blood pressure checkup at home.

High Blood Pressure Tests

When the heartbeats, a blood pressure check tests the strain within the arteries. You can get a blood pressure check as part of the appointment of a regular doctor, or as a high blood pressure monitoring (hypertension). Many people conduct their own blood pressure checks at home, for example, those with high blood pressure, so they can help monitor their health.

If you have been treated with high blood pressure (hypertension) or low blood pressure (hypotension), you can get more regular blood pressure checks.

Blood pressure monitoring is a routine component in most healthcare appointments.

The doctor may schedule different appointments for regular blood pressure tests and monitor for chronic health problems, including high blood pressure (hypertension), low blood pressure (hypotension), heart failure, etc.

To check for high blood pressure as a contributing factor for heart failure and stroke, you will get a blood pressure test done at least once every two years, beginning at age 18. Whether you are 40 years of age or older, even if you are 18 to 39 years of age with a higher risk of high blood pressure, remind the doctor every year for a test of blood pressure.

Unless there are potential risk factors for developing cardiac disease, such as being obese or having a family history of high blood pressure or heart disease, the doctor may suggest screening at a younger age. When you have ever been hospitalized with elevated or poor blood pressure, blood pressure checks will be performed more frequently.

The blood pressure is important information to the doctor, particularly though the doctor does not believe you have elevated or poor blood pressure as a chronic problem. This will provide details about your overall health.

The doctor may prescribe that you take blood pressure checks at home, in addition to routine blood pressure checks at a doctor's office. The home blood pressure devices are automatic and simple to use.

Medications to Treat High Blood Pressure

Angiotensin-converting enzyme (ACE) inhibitors

Some drugs such as lisinopril (Zestril), benazepril (Lotensin), captopril (Capoten), and others— tend to open blood vessels by preventing the production of a natural chemical that narrows the blood vessels. Persons with chronic kidney disease can benefit from using one of these drugs as an ACE inhibitor.

Angiotensin II receptor blockers (ARBs)

Some medicines tend to open blood vessels by preventing the activity of a natural chemical that narrows the blood flow, not the shape. Candesartan (Atacand), losartan (Cozaar), and others are included in ARB. Persons with chronic kidney disease can gain as one of their drugs from getting an ARB.

Calcium channel blockers

These medications like amlodipine (Norvasc), diltiazem (Cardizem, Tiazac, others), and so on help calm the blood vessel muscles. Your heart rate starts decreasing due to some of them. For older people, calcium channel blockers can function better than ACE inhibitors do alone.

Juice of Grapefruit reacts with some calcium channel blockers, increasing blood levels of the medication, and putting you at a higher risk of side effects. Speak to your pharmacist or doctor if you're concerned about interactions.

Additional medications

If you have trouble getting to your blood pressure level with concentrations of the above medicines, your doctor prescribes:

Alpha-blockers

Such medications reduce blood vessel nerve signals, reducing the influence of natural chemicals that widen the blood vessels. Alpha-blockers contain doxazosin (Cardura), Minipress (Prazosin), and others.

Alpha-beta blockers

Alpha-beta blockers delay the heartbeat to decrease the volume of blood that needs to be circulated into the arteries, in addition to minimizing nervous impulses through blood vessels. Blockers for the alpha-beta contain carvedilol (Coreg) and labetalol (Trandate).

Beta-blockers

Such medicines reduce the heart's pressure and expand the blood arteries, allowing the heart to pump more steadily and less violently. Acebutolol (Sectral), atenolol (Tenormin), and others are beta-blockers. Beta-blockers are typically not used as the only drug you are given, although they may be beneficial when paired with certain drugs for blood pressure.

Aldosterone antagonists

Examples include spironolactone (Aldactone) and inspire (Eplerenone). These medications inhibit the influence of natural chemicals and can lead to the accumulation of salt and sodium, which can add to high blood pressure.

Renin-inhibitors

Aliskiren (Tekturna) slows down renin development, an enzyme the kidneys generate that begins a series of chemical steps that raise blood pressure. Aliskiren functions by reducing the renin's ability to continue the cycle. You will not be taking aliskiren with ACE inhibitors or ARBs owing to a chance of severe problems, including stroke.

Vasodilators

Such medicines, including hydralazine and minoxidil, operate directly on the muscles in your artery walls, avoiding contracting the muscles and widening of the arteries.

Central-acting agents

Such medicines prohibit the brain from triggering the nervous system to raise your heart rate and narrow down the blood vessels. Clonidine (Catapres, Kapvay) and methyldopa are examples of this.

To minimize the number of regular doses of medication you need, your doctor can recommend a mixture of low-dose medicines instead of the larger doses of a single drug. In addition, two or three drugs for blood pressure are always more successful than one. This is often a matter of experience to determine the most appropriate treatment or a mixture of medications.

Resistant Hypertension (When Your Blood Pressure Is Very Hard To Control)

You could have resistant hypertension if the blood pressure stays stubbornly high after taking at least three separate forms of high blood pressure medications, one of which should normally be a diuretic.

People who have managed high blood pressure but at the same time require four separate forms of drugs are often known to have resistant hypertension to maintain such regulation. The possibility of high blood pressure being a contributing factor will usually be reconsidered.

Getting resistant hypertension does not really mean you can never reduce your blood pressure. In reality, once you and your doctor are willing to determine what's causing your constantly high blood pressure, there's a strong possibility you can reach that target with the aid of more successful care.

Diuretics (Water Pills)

Diuretics, also referred to as water pills, belong to a family of medications that extract extra salt and water from the body. They're also used to control elevated blood pressure, including hypertension. High blood pressure may be a factor leading to the progression of various types of heart disease.

Diuretics have proved to be successful in avoiding heart disease and stroke in multiple individuals when used as a medication for hypertension. Many foods and herbs also have diuretic effects, which make you urinate more frequently to consume excess fluids and sodium.

Thiazide diuretics tend to control hypertension by expanding the blood flow and eliminating any excess fluid from the body. Examples of thiazides contain metolazone (Zaroxolyn), indapamide (Lozol), and Microzide (Hydrochlorothiazide).

Loop diuretics eliminate extra fluid by allowing more urine to accumulate in the kidneys. These involve furosemide (Lasix), ethacrynic acid (Edecrin), and torsemide (Demadex), respectively.

Potassium-sparing diuretics allow the body to rid itself of salt and fluids. They do so, though, without triggering a shortage of potassium, a critical nutrient. Types of diuretics that conserve potassium contain triamterene (Dyrenium), eplerenone (Inspra), and spironolactone (Aldactone).

Increasing of the three forms of diuretic drug reduces the volume of sodium that you excrete by urination, which impacts different parts of the kidneys. The kidneys are the tubes by which the body flushes off contaminants and waste fluids. The treatment advises the liver while you are on a diuretic medicine that you want to get rid of more sodium. Blood attaches to the salt, which is absorbed through urination, providing you with a smaller amount of plasma. Reducing the amount of blood reduces the pace at which blood passes into the blood vessels, helping to reduce the blood pressure.

With water and sodium, thiazide and loop diuretics can also trigger you to lose potassium. Potassium is an essential mineral that preserves healthy fluid levels and controls the functioning of the heart and muscles. Your doctor can suggest taking a potassium supplement or consuming nutrient-rich foods to reduce low potassium levels.

Feeding stuffs high in potassium include:

- Bananas
- Avocados
- Raisins
- Beans
- Squash
- Mushrooms
- Potatoes
- Yogurt
- Fish

Diuretics that conserve potassium don't present as much a danger to the potassium rates. These are also not as successful in managing hypertension as the other forms of diuretic medications, and they are mostly used along with other medicines.

Thiazide diuretics are the main form of therapy for people with heart problems related to hypertension. The doctor may also adapt the prescription treatment to your specific health issues. The particular prescription may include a single pill or dose of more than one form of the diuretic agent.

Risks And Side Effects

Where used as indicated, diuretics are usually effective for most citizens. Enhanced urination is the most frequent side effect of diuretics. Depending on the type of diuretic you are taking, your potassium, glucose, and cholesterol levels can fluctuate. Your doctor can have blood checks performed during the care to assess the rates.

Other side effects may include:

- Headaches
- Dizziness or lightheadedness
- Difficulty sleeping
- Muscle weakness or cramping
- Increased thirst
- Irregular menstruation
- Difficulty achieving and maintaining an erection
- Conditions that cause swelling and pain in the joints of the foot

With time, adverse effects are expected to decrease. If you have unpleasant or persistent side effects when taking a diuretic, make sure to alert your doctor. Your doctor may change your dose, or you can turn to another form of the diuretic drug.

High Blood Pressure Treatment Follow-up

After beginning drug treatment for elevated blood pressure, you will visit a doctor at least once a month before you hit the target of blood pressure. Your doctor may test the amount of potassium in your blood once or twice a year (diuretics may lower this, and ACE inhibitors and ARBs may raise this) and other electrolytes and levels of BUN/creatinine (to test kidney health).

You will aim to visit the doctor for three or six months until the blood pressure target is met, based on whether you have any conditions, such as heart failure.

Chapter **2:** Risks Associated with High Blood Pressure

High blood pressure is a typical problem in which the blood's long-term force against the artery walls is strong enough to cause health issues, including heart disease potentially.

The blood pressure is measured by both the amount of blood pumped by your heart and the amount of blood flow resistance in your arteries.

High blood pressure can be present for many years without any symptoms. Even without the signs, the damage to the blood vessels and the heart can be observed. Uncontrolled hypertension (high blood pressure) raises the risk of severe health problems, like stroke and heart attack.

2.1 When to Worry About High Blood Pressure

A hypertensive (high blood pressure or HBP) problem arises when blood pressure with readings of 180/120 or higher rises rapidly and significantly.

The implications in this range of uncontrolled blood pressure can be severe, including:

- Stroke
- Loss of consciousness
- Memory loss
- Heart attack or heart failure
- Damage of Kidneys and eyes
- Kidneys Dysfunction
- Aortic dissection
- Unstable chest pain (Angina)
- Pulmonary edema
- Eclampsia

Some of the following symptoms may or may not be followed by an elevated reading:

- Nosebleeds
- Severe headache
- Severe anxiety
- Shortness of breath

Know the Two Types of High Blood Pressure Crisis to Watch For

There are two forms of hypertensive crises both need urgent treatment because it is essential to assess an effective course of action when determining the organ function early enough.

Hypertensive Urgency

If your blood pressure is higher than or equal to 180/120, wait around five minutes, and try again. When the second reading is just as high, and you don't experience any other related symptoms of target organ damage, such as chest pain, shortness of breath, back pain, numbness/weakness, vision disturbance, or speech trouble that will be called a hypertensive urgency. Your healthcare provider may just allow you to change or add drugs, but they rarely require hospitalization or any Hospital treatment.

Hypertensive Emergency

If the reading of your blood pressure is between the range of 180/120 or higher, and you are experiencing any other associated symptoms of target organ damage such as chest pain, shortness of breath, back pain, numbness/weakness, changes in your eyes vision, or difficulty in your speaking. This problem would be considered a hypertensive emergency. Do not wait to see if your pressure comes down on its own because you need special assistance.

Misconceptions About High Blood Pressure

Are you worried about the problem of high blood pressure in yourself, or your any family member, or your any friend? Or your concern is well-founded. If high blood pressure is left untreated, <u>high blood pressure</u>, then it also called hypertension, which can lead to a range of health problems, like <u>heart disease</u>, <u>stroke</u>, or kidney failure. Learning all about high blood pressure will help avoid harm to your health or even the health of anyone you love. You will start by knowing what, and what is not, true about this situation.

The following are some common misconceptions about <u>high blood pressure</u>:

- High Blood Pressure Isn't a Big Deal
- High Blood Pressure Can't Be Prevented
- It is completely Fine As Long As One Number Is Normal
- High Blood Pressure Is About Treatment

2.2 High Blood Pressure Leading To Heart Disease

The heart is influenced by many causes, which play a significant part in our health and medical conditions. The number one risk factor for cardiovascular disease is elevated blood pressure.

Typically, elevated blood pressure is asymptomatic. However, signs also appear after the illness has progressed so far as to damage organ functions. Many symptoms may include chest pain, swelling or discomfort, trouble breathing, epilepsy, numbness, speech problems (such as strokes), vomiting diarrhea, blurry vision, blood in the nose, and dullness.

Hypertensive Heart Disease

Hypertensive heart disease refers to high blood pressure heart problems.

The heart that functions under intense pressure trigger many cardiac problems. Hypertensive heart disease involves a respiratory arrest, heart muscle thickening, coronary artery disease, and other complications.

Hypertensive cardiovascular disease can cause severe health issues. This is the primary cause of blood pressure mortality.

Some Common Types of Hypertensive Heart Disease

Commonly, the heart problems associated with high blood pressure related to the heart's arteries and muscles.

The types of hypertensive heart disease include:

- Narrowing of the arteries
- Thickening and enlargement of the heart
- Complications

Who is a significant risk for hypertensive heart disease?

The major risk factor for hypertensive heart disease is high blood pressure, and your risk increases:

- If you're overweight
- If you don't exercise enough
- If you smoke
- If you eat food high in fat and cholesterol

Identifying the symptoms of hypertensive heart disease

Symptoms are depending on the severity of the condition and progression of the disease. Maybe you don't experience any symptoms, or you experienced the symptoms like:

- Pain in Chest
- Pressure or tightness in the chest
- Trouble in breathing
- Fatigue
- Pain in the back, neck, shoulders or arms
- Persistent Cough
- Loss of Appetite
- Ankle or Leg swelling

Testing and diagnosis of hypertensive heart disease
Your doctor will review your medical history, examine you physically, or run any lab tests to check your kidneys, sodium, potassium, and your blood count.
Some of the following tests may be used to help determine the cause of your symptoms:

- Electrocardiogram
- Echocardiogram
- Coronary angiography
- Exercise stress test
- The nuclear stress test examines the flow of blood into the heart

Treating Of Hypertensive Heart Disease
Hypertensive heart disease treatment depends on the severity of the illness, the age, and your medical background.
Medication
Medicines support the heart in many ways. The key aims are to avoid clotting the blood, increase blood supply, and reduce cholesterol levels in your body.
Some examples of the most common heart disease medications may include:

- Water pills to help lower blood pressure
- Nitrates to treat chest pain
- Statins to treat high cholesterol
- Calcium channel blockers and ace inhibitors to help lower blood pressure
- Aspirin to prevent blood clots

It's essential always to take all medications just precisely as prescribed.
Surgeries And Devices

In the more severe cases, you may require surgery to increase the heart's blood circulation. Your doctor may use a battery-operated system called a pacemaker in your chest if you need help controlling heart rate or rhythm. A pacemaker generates electrical pressure that allows the heart to contract. Pacemaker implantation is necessary and helpful when electrical muscle activation is too slow or absent.

2.3 High Cholesterol Levels Leading to High Blood Pressure

For a heart disease risk factor, you need to be aware of this factor. You have two options to make significant improvements in your life. Scientists also have shown that, when patients have more than one risk factor, such as elevated blood cholesterol and high blood pressure, this works together to increase the risk of heart failure.

Even if the cholesterol and blood pressure levels are just significantly elevated, if they both exist in your blood, they will combine and destroy the blood vessels and the heart more rapidly. If they are not managed, they ultimately set the stage for heart disease and stroke, along with other complications such as kidney failure and loss of vision.

When high blood cholesterol has already been diagnosed, monitor the blood pressure levels very seriously and regularly! Such two risk factors are very much in common. But if you know what's going on, you will win the fight for your health in your life.

Understanding High Cholesterol

When elevated cholesterol is diagnosed, it means that the blood cholesterol levels are higher than what is expected to be healthy. Cholesterol is a form of a fatty compound which use in your body for the processing and development of certain hormones, vitamin D, and healthy cells. We produce some in our bodies and get some from the food we consume.

Moreover, too much cholesterol can increase the risk of heart disease, heart disease, and stroke. The downside is that the extra fatty material will stick in the walls of your arteries if the cholesterol is high. Over time, this accumulation will build up a fatty layer, just like dirt and grime in a garden coat.

The fatty material gradually strengthens and develops a kind of inflexible layer that destroying the arteries. They are close and dense, and the blood is not as quickly flowing into them as it used to be.

The greatest risk is that the blood vessel will obstruct blood supply, leading to serious heart problems.

How High Cholesterol Can Lead To High Blood Pressure

If elevated blood cholesterol is detected, you could take medications to control it, so you might have changed your diet spontaneously to help reduce your cholesterol rates.

In the meantime, keeping an eye on your blood pressure is important. People with elevated blood cholesterol frequently often end up with high blood pressure.

2.4 Effects of Hypertension on Daily Life

High blood pressure has no symptoms unless you begin to experience complications in your body. That's why it's important to monitor your blood pressure regularly.

Following are some effects of hypertension on the body:

Circulatory System

High blood pressure damage starts low and increases over time. The more it goes undiagnosed or untreated, the more serious the risks are.

The blood vessels and large arteries transport blood all over the body and provide it with vital tissue and organ. As the blood pressure rises, it begins to damage the walls of the artery.

Damage starts as small tears. As these tears continue to form in the bloodstream, harmful cholesterol circulating in the blood begins to bind to the tissues. Increasingly, cholesterol accumulates in the lungs, raising the artery. Less blood can pass through.

When a blocked artery cannot move the appropriate volume of blood, it can damage the tissue or organ it will enter. It can mean chest pressure, pulse, or a heart attack.

The heart still works better, but with high blood pressure and narrowed arteries, it is less successful. The extra work will ultimately lead to an inflated left ventricle that is the part of the heart that pumps blood into the body. It further raises the chance of a heart attack.

Cardiac failure occurs when the heart is so sluggish, hypertensive, or heart attacks that it stops circulating blood effectively through the body

Symptoms Of Heart Failure May Include:

- Shortness of the breath
- Trouble in breathing
- Swelling of the feet, ankles, legs, or in the abdomen
- Tired feeling

High blood pressure can also contribute to the development of a bulge in the affected arteries. That is referred to as an aneurysm. The bulge grows broader and deeper and sometimes is not noticed until it causes discomfort when it presses or explodes against some part of the body.

If in one of the major arteries, a ruptured aneurysm can be fatal. This can occur anywhere in the body.

The Skeletal System

High blood pressure in the body may cause bone loss, called osteoporosis, by increasing the amount of calcium your body may get rid of when you urinate. Women that have already experienced menopause may especially at risk.

Osteoporosis weakens the muscles, which makes the fractures and the breaks easier to occur.

The Respiratory System

Like the heart and brain, in the lungs, arteries can also damage and block. It's termed as pulmonary embolism when an artery that brings blood to the lungs is blocked. To track that, it's really dangerous and necessary and requires urgent medical attention. An aneurysm can occur in the lungs, too.

Sleep Disorder

Sleep apnea is a type of sleep disorder that causes loud snoring and interruptions in breathing during sleep. People with sleep apnea, when waking up in the after sleep, still do not feel rested. Research has related the disorder to high blood pressure as high blood pressure is also present in many people diagnosed with sleep apnea.

The Reproductive System

In arousal, sex organs use extra blood flow. Sexual dysfunction can occur in the body when hypertension (high blood pressure) causes many blockages to the blood vessels, which leads to the body's sexual organs.

Males may have a hard risk to getting and maintaining an erection, and women might experience:

- Decreased arousal
- Vaginal dryness
- Trouble having an orgasm

Urinary System

Kidneys help to remove waste from the blood, regulate blood volume and pressure, and filter waste out through urine. Kidneys require healthy blood vessels for this to be done well.

High blood pressure can damage smaller blood vessels within your kidneys and larger vessels leading to the kidneys. Over time this damage always prevents the kidneys from properly doing their work. This is known as kidney disease and can result in failure. Hypertension (High blood pressure) is the most critical cause of kidney failure. Patients with kidney disease are no longer able to expel waste from their organs so that they may require either dialysis or a transplant.

Damage The Kidneys

Kidneys remove the blood's excess fluid and waste, a mechanism that includes safe blood vessels. High blood pressure can cause damage to the blood vessels, which can lead to the kidneys. In addition to high blood pressure, having diabetes will make harm worse.

High blood pressure causing kidney issues include:

- Kidney Scarring (Glomerulosclerosis)
- Kidney failure

Damage to Eyes

High blood pressure damages the tiny, delicate blood vessels that work to supply blood to your eyes which causing the damage of eyes:

Damages of eyes, including:

- Damage to your retina (retinopathy)
- Fluid buildup under the retina (choroidopathy)
- Nerve damage (optic neuropathy)

High Blood Pressure Emergencies

Typically, high blood pressure is a lifelong disease that causes harm over the years. But often blood pressure increases so quickly and so significantly that it is a medical emergency, sometimes needs hospitalization for proper recovery.

In such situations, hypertension (high blood pressure) can cause:

- Loss of Memory
- Changes in Personality
- Trouble in concentration
- A progressive loss of consciousness or Irritability

- Strokes
- Damage to the body's main artery
- Pain in Chest
- Heart attack
- All of the sudden impaired pumping of your heart, leading to fluid backup in the lungs resulting in the shortness of breath
- Sudden loss of the kidney function
- Pregnancy complications
- Blindness

Effects Of Hypertension On Mind

Hypertension is a dysfunction of the circulatory system. All parts of the body are dependent on circulation, and several organs suffer from the untreated hypertension effect. One of the highest-risk organs is the brain.

Blood pressure is the vital force that drives blood that is rich in oxygen to all parts of your body. Your heart is the force-generating pump, and your arteries are the pathways that contain and circulate the blood.

The height of your blood pressure is measured by how deeply the main pumping chamber of your heart, the left ventricle, contracts, and the diameter and hardness of your arteries. In effect, a vast number of genetic, biochemical, physiological, neurological, psychological, and lifestyle factors affect your heart and arteries, which decide your blood pressure. Because these factors are so diverse and nuanced, the blood pressure during the course of the day can vary from minute to minute and hour to hour, not to mention the smaller changes that occur over a lifetime.

Blood pressure is composed of two sections. The greater number is called the systolic blood pressure, which is measured when your heart is pumping blood into your arteries; the lower number is the diastolic blood pressure, which is reported while your heart is relaxing and blood is refilling in it between beats. Both figures are measured into millimeters of mercury (mm Hg), a vestige of the column of mercury used more than 100 years ago in the first pressure manometers. Usually, the higher number is first reported; systolic pressure of 110 mm Hg and a diastolic pressure of 70 mm Hg will be written as 110/70 and pronounced "110 over 70." In adults, normal blood pressure indicates that you have less than 120/80 readings. The systolic blood pressure between 120 and 129 is defined as high blood pressure according to the current guidelines.

Stage 1 high blood pressure (a hypertension diagnosis) is now between 130 and 139 systolic, or between 80 and 89 diastolic (the lowest number). Level 2 of elevated blood pressure is usually 140 systolic or 90 diastolic or higher.

Indeed, hypertension is extremely consequential; it contributes to one in six deaths in adults. Hypertension is known as a cardiovascular disease because it affects the heart and blood vessels. However, since arteries are essential to the health of all our organs, hypertension is a multisystem disease. For many cases, the most damaging effect of hypertension does not occur on the heart but the eyes, kidneys, and, most probably, the brain.

Stroke

There are two main stroke forms, ischemic and hemorrhagic. Hemorrhagic strokes are less severe but also cause the most dramatic symptoms. These arise when a blood vessel bursts into the brain, spilling blood into the brain or the fluid surrounding it.

Ischemic strokes, which account for nearly 87 percent of all strokes, occur when a clot blocks an artery that provides blood to the brain. This can occur in two forms. During a thrombotic stroke, the clot inside the brain itself occurs in a diseased artery. The clot grows out of the brain in an embolic stroke, then breaks free, and is transported by the blood to the brain, at which it places in a previously healthy artery. Most emboli occur in carotid artery or aorta on atherosclerotic plaques, or in the heart itself.

Each of these big stroke forms features a milder counterpart. While it is difficult to ignore the large hemorrhagic strokes, MRI studies show that small microbleeds are much more usual. Similarly, because of their small size, many people have tiny ischemic strokes, which are known as lacunar strokes. Although it is unlikely that a simple micro bleed or lacunar stroke would trigger symptoms, a variety of such incidents may cause significant problems, including memory loss or cognitive dysfunctions. More than 13 million people have had one or more of those "silent" strokes that are particularly common in people who are over 60, especially if they have hypertension, according to a study.

Types of Stroke

- Hemorrhagic stroke
- Subarachnoid hemorrhage
- Intracerebral hemorrhage
- Ischemic stroke
- Embolic stroke
- Thrombotic stroke

Chapter 3: Treating High Blood Pressure Naturally With Diet

They are changing the diet will probably lower hypertension. Research has shown that some foods can reduce blood pressure, both rapidly and in the long term.

High blood pressure impacts 1 in 3 people worldwide. Drugs, dietary improvements, and other behavioral adjustments may lower elevated blood pressure without reducing the risk of related conditions. Getting high blood pressure raises the possibility of heart attack, stroke, and kidney disease.

3.1 Foods That Lower Blood Pressure

There are certain foods and beverages that will normally lower blood pressure.

Natural Foods

Many diets may help lower high blood pressure and will provide medical evidence. Several studies have shown certain diets can minimize high blood pressure. Just take a look at which products work and how they can be integrated into a balanced diet.

Berries

Blueberries and strawberries produce antioxidant compounds, a form of flavonoid called anthocyanins. We observed that people with the largest consumption of anthocyanins, mainly from blueberries and strawberries, have an 8% decrease in the incidence of high blood pressure compared with those with small consumption of anthocyanin. Enjoy berries between meals as a snack or sweet treat, or add to the smoothies and oatmeal.

Bananas

Bananas include plenty of potassium, a mineral that plays a vital role in hypertension management. One medium-sized banana has about 422 milligrams of potassium in it.

Potassium decreases the influence of sodium and soothes discomfort in the walls of the blood vessels, according to the study. Adults will strive for a maximum intake of 4,700 milligrams (mg) of potassium.

Certain foods which are high in potassium include:

- Avocado
- Cantaloupe And Honeydew Melon
- Halibut
- Mushrooms
- Sweet Potatoes
- Tomatoes
- Tuna
- Beans

People who have kidney disease can speak about potassium with their physicians since too much intake of potassium can be dangerous.

Beets

Drinking beet juice will reduce short-and long-term blood pressure. Researchers found that consuming red beet juice resulted in lower blood pressure in people with hypertension who consumed about 1 cup of juice for four weeks every day. Within 24 hours, the researchers found a few beneficial results.

Those who consumed 1 cup of the beet juice a day had an average reduction in blood pressure of approximately 8/4 millimeters of mercury (mm Hg). This move has put the blood pressure into the usual range. A standard blood pressure drug lowers concentrations by 9/5 mm Hg on average.

The researchers proposed that a decrease in blood pressure was caused by elevated amounts of inorganic nitrate from beets. Having a glass of beet juice each day will help introduce beets to salads or serve the veggies as a nutritious side dish.

Dark Chocolate

This delicious treat could bring down blood pressure. The analysis shows that cocoa-rich chocolate in humans with hypertension or prehypertension lowers blood pressure.

Select high-quality chocolate that includes at least 70 percent of cocoa and eat a single slice or one portion that weighs around 1 ounce a day.

Kiwis

According to the findings of one study, a daily serving of kiwi will reduce blood pressure in people with slightly elevated levels. The researchers contrasted apple and kiwi influences on people with mildly elevated blood pressure.

They noticed that consuming three kiwis a day for eight weeks resulted in a larger decrease in both systolic and diastolic blood pressure, relative to consuming one apple a day for the same duration. The researchers believe the decline has been triggered by the bioactive compounds in kiwis.

Kiwis are also high in vitamin C, which can substantially increase blood pressure levels in people who have been eating about 500 mg of vitamin regularly for around eight weeks. Kiwis can conveniently be added to lunches or smoothies too.

Watermelon

Watermelons contain the amino acid called coralline, which may better treat hypertension.

Coralline makes the body generate nitric oxide, a substance that relaxes blood vessels and promotes arterial flexibility. Such results improve blood pressure and may reduce hypertension. In one test, ankles and brachial arteries demonstrated decreased blood pressure in adults with obesity and prehypertension, or moderate hypertension who took watermelon extract. The brachial artery in the upper arm is the primary artery.

Researchers have also observed that animals with a watermelon saturated diet have a stronger cardiac function. In one test, mice who consumed a watermelon juice solution had a 50 percent lower plaque in their vessels than the control group.

To maximize the consumption of watermelon, add the fruit to the salads and smoothies or drink it in a cold broth of watermelon.

Oats

Oats produce a form of fiber named beta-glycan that can lower cholesterol rates in the blood. According to some studies, beta-glycan often may reduce blood pressure.

A study of 28 studies found that a higher intake of beta-glycan fiber may lower the blood pressure, both systolic and diastolic. Barley includes fiber as well.

Begin the day off with just a bowl of oatmeal, or using rolled oats to give meat or vegetarian burger patties a crunch instead of breadcrumbs.

Leafy Green Vegetables

Green leafy vegetables are high in nitrates, which help with blood pressure control. Some evidence shows that consuming 1–2 portions of vegetables high in nitrate per day will minimize hypertension for approximately 24 hours.

Examples of leafy greens include:

- Cabbage
- Collard Greens
- Fennel
- Kale Lettuce
- Mustard Greens
- Spinach
- Swiss Chard

Stir spinach into curries and stews to enjoy a full dose of green veggies, sauté Swiss chard with garlic for a savory side dish, or cook a batch of kale chips.

Garlic

Garlic is a safe product and is both antibiotic and antifungal. The main active component is also blamed for the safety advantages linked with it.

Some work indicates that garlic increases nitric oxide output in the body, which helps relax the smooth muscles and dilate the blood vessels. Hypertension may be reduced by certain improvements.

One research recorded that in hypertensive men, garlic extract lowered the systolic and diastolic blood pressure.

Garlic will improve several tasty dishes, including stir-fries, soups, and omelets. Use garlic rather than salt may help improve cardiac health.

Fermented Foods

Fermented products are abundant in probiotics, good bacteria that play a significant role in preserving well-being in the stomach. Eating probiotics could have a moderate impact on high blood pressure, a study has found.

More enhanced results identified by the researchers while study participants were consuming:

- Multiple Species Of Probiotic Bacteria
- Probiotics Regularly For More Than Eight Weeks
- At Least 100 Billion Colony-Forming Units A Day
- Fermented Foods To Add To The Diet Include:
- Natural Yogurt
- Kimchee
- Apple Cider Vinegar
- Miso
- Tempeh

Lentils and Other Pulses

Lentils are favorite in many diets worldwide, because they are an ideal vegetarian protein and fiber source. Scientists who researched the impact of a pulses-rich diet reported reduced blood pressure and cholesterol rates. A minimum of 30% of the individual's diet contained beans, peas, lentils, and chickpeas.

Lentils are rather powerful and versatile. Most consumers are using them as a healthy substitute for haunted beef by incorporating bulk to salads and soups.

Natural Yogurt

The researchers have confirmed yogurt can reduce women's risk of high blood pressure.

The researchers observed that middle-aged women who ingested five or more portions of yogurt per week for 18–30 years, showed a 20 percent decrease in the incidence of hypertension relative to women of comparable age who barely eat yogurt.

The males in the research did not seem to have the same advantages, but their levels of yogurt seemed to be larger.

Unsweetened yogurts, such as regular or Greek yogurts, appear to benefit more. Enjoy them for a balanced snack or meal with berries, nuts, or seeds.

Pomegranates

Drinking 1 cup of pomegranate juice every day for 28 days will, according to a study's results, minimize high blood pressure in the short term. The researchers related the influence on the antioxidant content of the fruits.

Although you may appreciate pomegranates whole, some people choose the extracts. Try to ensure that there is no additional sugar when purchasing pre-packaged pomegranate juice.

Cinnamon

Cinnamon may also tend to relieve blood pressure in the short term, at least.

A three-study review found that cinnamon reduced short-term systolic blood pressure by 5.39 mm Hg and diastolic blood pressure by 2.6 mm Hg. There is still a need for further study.

Apply cinnamon to the diet as an alternative to sugar by sprinkling it over oatmeal or freshly cut berries. Cinnamon can be bought in several different ways.

Pistachios

Pistachios are healthy nuts that can lower hypertension. One research indicated that a moderate-fat diet, including pistachio nuts, could reduce blood pressure during periods of stress. That may be because the tightness of blood vessels is diminished by a compound in the nuts. Many experiments also have shown a strong influence on other nuts, such as almonds. Snack on simple pistachios, add them in salads, or blend them in pesos. Unsalted nuts are safer.

Water Intake (Reducing Dehydration)

Dehydration occurs anytime when there isn't enough water in the body. Not consuming enough water or losing more liquid than you can absorb will also contribute to dehydration.

Dehydration can be severe. These may lead to life-threatening risks, such as heat-related illnesses and kidney issues if left unchecked. In addition, dehydration can potentially cause hazardous changes in blood pressure.

How Does Dehydration Affect Your Blood Pressure?

Blood pressure is the stress generated by the blood against the lining of your arteries and veins. Dehydration will influence your blood flow and trigger your blood pressure to rise or go down. Let's dig into why this occurs more closely.

Dehydration and Low Blood Pressure

Low blood pressure occurs anytime the measurement of the blood pressure is less than 90/60 mm Hg. Because of the reduction of blood flow, dehydration may produce low blood pressure.

The blood pressure is the sum of fluids in the blood vessels that are moving. Maintaining a regular blood flow is important in order for the blood to reach all of the body's tissues properly.

Your blood volume can decrease when you're very dehydrated, resulting in a drop in blood pressure.

When blood pressure decreases so far, the muscles do not receive the oxygen and nutrients that they need. You might be slipping into shock, possibly.

Dehydration and High Blood Pressure

High blood pressure occurs whether you get a 140 mm Hg or higher systolic (top number) reading, or a 90 mm Hg or higher diastolic reading.

Dehydration was correlated with high blood pressure. Research into this subject is, however, restricted. In order to investigate the relation, more work is needed.

While further work is required, it is still worth remembering that dehydration due to the activity of a hormone called vasopressin can contribute to elevated blood pressure.

Vasopressin is secreted when your blood produces a large number of solutes (or sodium level), or when your blood pressure is low. This will happen when you lack too much fluid.

In addition, the kidneys reabsorb water while you're dehydrated, as opposed to losing it in the urine. Large amounts of vasopressin can also induce constriction of the blood vessels. This may contribute to higher blood pressure.

Other Symptoms of Dehydration

There are other symptoms of dehydration to look out for besides fluctuation in blood pressure.

You'll also experience the signs until you realize you've experienced a rise in blood pressure.

Such symptoms are:

- Thirst
- Dry Mouth
- Urinating Less Often
- Urine That's Dark In Color
- Feeling Tired or Fatigued
- Lightheadedness or Dizziness
- Confusion

Causes of Dehydration

There are other potential reasons for deficiency apart from not drinking enough water. These may include:

- Illness: High fever can cause dehydration. In addition, vomiting and diarrhea may contribute to significant fluid and electrolyte depletion.

- Extra sweating: If you sweat, the energy is lost. There may be an uptick in sweating in hot weather, during training, even whether you're ill with a fever.
- Often urinating: You will waste fluids through urination, too. Drugs such as diuretics, chronic disorders such as asthma, and the intake of alcohol may also induce more regular urination.

The trick to avoiding dehydration is to ensure that you are getting in enough liquids every day. But just how much amount of water or other fluids are you expected to get in a day?

Recommendations for daily fluid can rely on many factors, including:

- Age
- Sex
- Weight
- Overall health
- Weather conditions
- Activity level
- Pregnancy or breastfeeding
- A healthy goal for this is to consume at least eight glasses of water per day

You should remain hydrated by drinking following fluids if you consider it hard to drink pure water:

- Water infused with slices of fruit, like lemon or cucumber
- Sugar-free sparkling water
- Smoothies made with fruits and vegetables
- Decaffeinated herbal tea
- Milk
- **Low sodium soups**

Remember also that some of the food sources, especially fruits and vegetables, will provide you water.

Alternatively, adopt the following guidelines to help keep yourself hydrated:

- Always drink when you are thirsty. Feeling hungry is the reason the body informs you they need more fluids.
- Try to consume extra fluids while you are overly busy, in extreme weather, or recovering from fatigue, vomiting, or diarrhea.
- Take a glass of water with you when you go through your everyday job. This means you're still going to have water on deck.
- Use water rather than soft drinks, caffeine drinks, sweetened drinks, or alcoholic beverages.

Nutrients

The following are some nutrients that have been proven helpful in reducing blood pressure.

- Potassium-rich foods
- Foods with high fiber
- Magnesium-rich foods

Potassium-Rich Foods

Foods rich in potassium are essential for controlling high blood pressure (HBP or hypertension) since potassium decreases sodium effects. The more you ingest potassium, the more sodium you remove in the urine. Potassium also helps relieve strain in the walls of the bloodstream, which can reduce blood pressure much more.

It's advised to improve potassium by diet in adults with blood pressure over 120/80 who are otherwise healthy. Potassium may be dangerous in those with kidney failure; any illness is influencing how potassium is treated by the body or anyone on other drugs. Deciding how to take extra potassium with the doctor will be discussed.

Potassium and Your Diet

For an average adult, the recommended intake of potassium is 4,700 milligrams (mg) per day.

Some of the DASH (Dietary Approaches to Stop Hypertension) diet components: nuts, beans, fat-free or low-fat (1 percent) dairy products and seafood are healthy natural potassium sources. For instance, there is around 420 mg of potassium in a medium banana, and 475 mg in a half cup of pure mashed sweet potato.

Some other potassium-rich foods include:

- Apricots and apricot juice
- Avocados
- Cantaloupe and honeydew melon
- Fat-free or low-fat (1 percent) milk
- Fat-free yogurt
- Grapefruit and grapefruit juice (talk to your healthcare provider if you're taking a cholesterol-lowering drug)
- Greens
- Halibut
- Lima beans
- Molasses
- Mushrooms
- Oranges and orange juice
- Peas
- Potatoes
- Prunes and prune juice
- Raisins and dates
- Spinach
- Tomatoes, tomato juice, and tomato sauce
- Tuna

While potassium can diminish the effects of sodium on blood pressure, consuming more potassium should also be coupled with your attempts to break up the excess salt and improve other healthier eating and lifestyle habits.

For people with kidney problems, too much potassium may be dangerous. When your blood is less capable of removing potassium from your kidneys, too much potassium can build up.

Sometimes there aren't many signs of elevated potassium (hyperkalemia), like excessive blood pressure. Feeling sick to the stomach will result in a small, slow, or erratic heartbeat and fainting with higher potassium rates.

Consult with a health care doctor before consuming some potassium replacement over the countered. When seeking salt replacements, you can always ask the doctor who will increase potassium in patients with other health problems and others who take high blood pressure ACE inhibitors.

High Fiber Foods

Fiber essentially makes you poop. When you choose to subscribe to a diet that is rich in processed foods and minimal in plant-based ingredients, you are more prone to experience stomach problems — including hunger.

You receive fiber from vegetables since parts of certain products are not actually digestible to the body. Then it pushes certain pieces to be removed into the digestive tract, bringing other items around the way with it.

Research has shown that consuming enough fiber regularly will contribute to reducing high blood pressure and eliminate it. Scientists aren't entirely sure why that is, although, among other reasons, it undoubtedly has something to do with the role of fiber in weight gain and blood sugar.

Those who consume the required dietary fiber do report reduced cholesterol, regular bowel motions, good digestive safety, and lower blood sugar. It's much more probable that if you regularly consume sufficiently high fiber meals, you would be able to achieve and sustain a healthier weight.

Experts suggest eating:

- 14 grams of fibers for every 1,000 calories you ingest in a day
- 25 grams of fiber for women of age between 18 to 50; 21 grams for women over 50
- For men, 30-38 grams of fiber.

Technically, fiber may be ingested in two ways: by fiber tablets, and thorough cooking.

Can You Take A Fiber Supplement With High Blood Pressure?

You may buy online or in-store fiber supplements, and there are various styles. When cooking, you can take a pill or apply some powder to your meal. What medicine you want always depends on the advice of your doctor and the reason you would like to take it. Older reports have shown that supplementing the fiber may help regulate blood pressure. So you should be allowed to use a fiber pill or some form of medication to improve your dose as long as you speak with the doctor to learn which remedy to use, how often, and how much you can. You would also speak to a doctor regarding any drugs you are contemplating taking because they conflict with the medicines you have been given for any health conditions.

Nonetheless, high-fiber diets should still be the best and most effective method of having the desired fiber per day. Supplements aren't tightly monitored; you don't really realize what's in them. And in certain instances, in addition to nutrients, food is a healthier option for added health benefits. It's beneficial for your general health to learn to eat fruits and vegetables, not just your weight or blood pressure.

Magnesium-Rich Foods

Magnesium is a mineral that occurs naturally and is important for the proper functioning of the human body. In addition, the magnesium directly depends on more than 300 biochemical processes. While magnesium is the fourth most common mineral in the human body, in practice, very little circulates in the blood or other tissues. Instead, much magnesium store on the body is stored away in our bones ' strong outer layer. Magnesium is processed from the foods we consume, it is consumed in the small intestine, and large amounts are excreted by the kidneys.

There has been growing concern in the potential function that magnesium can have in avoiding and treating diseases such as high blood pressure and cardiovascular disease over the last few years.

Can Magnesium Prevent High Blood Pressure?

One research finds evidence that seems to suggest magnesium plays a significant role in controlling blood pressure. In addition, a variety of other researchers have looked at specific dietary variables and how they relate to high blood pressure reduction. These tests have shown that magnesium-rich diets also seem to have a beneficial effect and that individuals with magnesium-rich diets tend to experience high blood pressure at a slower pace.

Oral Magnesium Supplements

No evidence was sufficient to support the argument that oral magnesium supplements provide the same benefits as a diet high in magnesium. While magnesium can be useful, as with other minerals, it may be the case that the way you get magnesium is just as essential as the magnesium itself. The human body, in other terms, is really effective at digesting organic food and consuming the vitamins and minerals that it provides.

On the other side, it does not seem that the human body is very effective at obtaining any nutritional value from various forms of dietary supplements. The best way to receive the required regular magnesium intake (RDA) is from natural food sources. The male RDA is about 420 mg for stable adults and the female RDA is around 320 mg or 360 mg for maternity.

Dietary Sources of Magnesium

Magnesium is present in a large variety of safe, inexpensive products. Fish and nuts are particularly abundant in minerals, 1 ounce (a tiny handful) of almonds produces around 80 mg of magnesium. Potatoes, carrots, and low-fat dairy foods, and other vegetables such as spinach, are also strong sources of magnesium like.

- Cooked white fish, 3oz: 90mg
- Cashews, 1oz: 75mg
- Medium baked potato: 50mg
- Plain low-fat yogurt, 8oz: 45mg

- Medium banana: 30mg
- Ready-to-eat pudding, 4oz: 24mg

Additionally, each of these foods is a healthy source of potassium and calcium, which helps to prevent and control high blood pressure. A basic thumb rule for consuming a balanced diet involves enjoying foods that come in several different colors. Red onions, green peppers, yellow bananas, white potatoes, etc.

Herbs

Most people often struggle with hypertension. Quick half of American people may soon be classified as having elevated blood pressure thanks to new improvements in recommendations. Doctors suggest making dietary adjustments and medicine for managing the disorder.

When, for medicinal purposes, you are talking about seeking plants, whether it's the entire herb or a substitute, first speak to the doctor. Low blood pressure experts actually do not prescribe medications daily. Some herbs may cause adverse side effects or interact with other drugs, particularly in large quantities.

Read on for more detail on the herbs and the study surrounding them.

Basil

Basil is a tasty herb, ideally adapted for a range of foods. It can help to reduce blood pressure, too. Basil extract has been shown to reduce blood pressure in, but only momentarily. The chemicals contained in basil can block some substances which tighten the blood vessels. It could result in a reduction of blood pressure. We need further research.

It's easy to add fresh basil to your diet, and it definitely can't harm. Hold in your kitchen garden a little herb pot and apply the fresh leaves to kinds of pasta, soups, salads, and casseroles.

Cinnamon

Cinnamon is another tasty spice that takes no work to be used in your regular diet, which will reduce your blood pressure numbers.

One research indicated that cinnamon extract had both reduced sudden-onset and chronic high blood pressure. The drug was given intravenously nevertheless. It's unclear if orally ingested cinnamon is successful, too.

You should add more cinnamon to your diet by sprinkling it on your cereal, oatmeal, and even on your coffee. Cinnamon at dinner improves the stir-fries, curries, and stews taste.

Cardamom

Cardamom is a seasoning that originates in India and is often used in South Asian cuisine. A global study of 20 individuals studying cardamom's health effects showed that subjects with elevated blood pressure reported substantial decreases in their blood pressure levels following 12 weeks of consuming 1.5 grams of cardamom powder twice every day. With a different taste and a potential beneficial health advantage, you should use cardamom seeds or powder in seasoning mixes, soups, and stews, and even boiled products.

Flaxseed

Flaxseed is high in omega-3 fatty acids, which has been shown to reduce blood pressure in several tests. A new study recommended for more than 12 weeks taking 30–50 grams of whole or ground seeds a day to get the maximum benefits. Flaxseed can defend against coronary atherosclerotic disease by reducing serum cholesterol, increasing glucose tolerance, and serving as an antioxidant.

Many items that contain flaxseed can be bought, but a safer choice is to buy whole or ground flaxseed and apply it to your homemade meals. The greatest thing regarding flaxseed is that it can be mixed from soups and smoothies and baked goods into nearly any bowl. The storing of flax seed in your freezer can help to preserve optimum potency.

Garlic

This seasoning pungent will do more than just taste your food and spoil your breath. Garlic could have the potential to reduce the blood pressure by trying to raise a compound in the body recognized as nitric oxide that will calm and dilate the blood vessels. This helps blood to circulate more naturally and decreases blood pressure.

A variety of your favorite dishes may be fresh garlic incorporated. If the taste is too intense for you, first roast on the garlic. And if you really can't eat the things, in supplement form, you can get garlic.

Ginger

Ginger can help in managing blood pressure. It has been shown in research to increase blood supply and calm the muscles around the blood vessels, thus reducing blood pressure. Until now, clinical experiments have been inconclusive. Ginger is a popular component widely used in Asian dishes, which may also be added to desserts or drinks. Chop, slim or grate fresh ginger into stir-fries, soups, and vegetable or noodle dishes, or apply to sweets or tea for a soothing taste.

Hawthorn

Hawthorn is a high blood pressure herbal treatment, used for thousands of years in ancient Chinese medicines. H In mice, hawthorn extracts tend to have a whole range of cardiovascular safety effects, including helping to reduce blood pressure, avoiding heart hardening, and reducing cholesterol. You may take hawthorn as a tablet, as an extract of liquid or as tea.

Celery Seed

Celery seeds are herbs that are used to spice soups, stews, casseroles, and other savory items. Celery has long been used in China for the treatment of hypertension, and studies have proven it to be successful. You should only use the seeds, or you could just juice the whole herb. Celery can also be a diuretic, demonstrating its impact on blood pressure. Researchers think a number of celery compounds may play a part in reducing blood pressure. There is also a requirement for human research.

French Lavender

Lavender's stunning, perfume-like fragrance is not the only useful feature of the herb. Extracts of lavender have been shown to minimize heart rate and blood pressure. While not many people think that lavender can be used as a cooking herb, the flowers can be used in baked foods. You should use **the leaves the same way you can use the rosemary.**

3.2 List of Foods to Avoid In High Blood Pressure

When you become diagnosed with hypertension, the healthcare professional may instruct you about how to treat it, whether by improvements of lifestyle, such as beginning the workout regimen or eating healthier, and/or treatment. Nonetheless, treating hypertensive patients has taught that it can be difficult to maintain control of what to consume and what to stop. To help you get going, here's a rundown of 10 foods and beverages that you need to be vigilant with or avoid to help reduce your blood pressure.

Table Salt

Salt is one of the most dangerous foods for people with high blood pressure, so ensuring you don't consume too much of it is crucial. It may sound fairly straightforward, but salt is hard to escape, really. Many people love to apply salt to their food like me. After all, it is a simple way to improve every dish's taste profile. This may even be tough to predict whether the products contain a lot of salt.

Researchers also have shown that rising salt consumption to 1,500 mg a day (less than half a teaspoon) will help lower approximately five mmHg of systolic blood pressure.

When you're having trouble keeping salt out of food, then concentrate on other foods that will help make the dishes taste great. That takes us to the next component.

Sauces and Condiments

If told to skip table salt, people sometimes opt for condiments such as ketchup, steak sauce, soy sauce, or salad dressings instead. But if you glance at their ingredients, you'll soon find they've got a lot of salt in them too! For Italian dishes, both red and white sauces have loads of salt, and so does gravy. It is named as "hidden salt." One bit of advice will be to use herbs and spices, to consider some varieties besides "salty."

Canned Foods

Most canned tomatoes, soups, and other nutritional items are cooked to taste and protect the nutrition with plenty of salt. Patients are always advised to stop such foods whenever necessary, preferring new veggies or low-salt soups instead. When you choose to use canned vegetables, you should purchase the "no salt applied" form or rinse the vegetables and get rid of the extra salt before cooking. Similarly, canned tuna is also heavy in salt, so try to give it a rinse too.

Processed Foods

Most packaged products contain tons of salt, just as canned veggies and soups. It covers several frozen foods, such as pizzas and frozen meals. The best recommendation here is to skip newly made dishes in lieu of such foods. Alternatively, search for low-salt alternatively low-sodium varieties if you don't have any other options. Many manufacturers consider the goods safer for those with asthma and heart failure.

Unhealthy Snacks

Everybody enjoys mumming in meals or at the end of the day on treats. When you glance at the snack lane, though, what do you think? Chips, biscuits, crackers, jerky, almonds, they all have loads of salt in them! In reality, that makes snacks so addictive is their salt, fat, and sugar. Popular chip flavorings such as country, salt and vinegar, bacon, and barbecue are all rich in salt, for instance. Search for varieties with minimal to no added salt. One choice is to purchase regular popcorn and incorporate your own seasoning, and there's no reason to think about salt at all.

Cured Meats

Chicken, bacon, and meats are frequently cooked by boiling them in saltwater and hot brine wash. Although cured meats may be absolutely wonderful, preventing them is better. Look out anytime you go out to eat and particularly when you're making a sandwich, especially during the holidays. Sandwiches are very strong in salt as they all have salt in their pasta, cheese, condiments, and meat. Getting more than 2,000 mg of salt for one sub or sandwich is relatively straightforward.

Pickled Foods

Pickled foods, including cured meats, bear a lot of salt too. Pickling is a method in which food remains in a salt solution (to destroy harmful bacteria) and other flavoring agents. Therefore pickled products are also heavy in salt. If your blood pressure troubles you, stop consuming pickles or other pickled items such as kimchee and sauerkraut, or at thoroughly rinse them before consuming to get rid of any of the salt.

Alcohol

An alcoholic beverage may marginally increase your blood pressure, but if you consume too much, your blood pressure can rise rapidly. Cutting back to normal rates will reduce blood pressure by around four mmHg for people who consume alcohol on a regular or semi-daily basis. The practitioners advise no more than one or two beverages a day for men and no more than one drink a day for women.

Caffeine

Coffee, tea, and energy drinks usually come with caffeine, which may raise blood pressure. Caffeine is not necessarily a concern for those with high blood pressure, so if you have hypertension, it is advised that you restrict the consumption of caffeine and then select decaf or half-cuffed coffee or caffeine-free teas.

High-Fat Foods

Although high-fat diets do not increase the blood pressure explicitly, they can cause other complications, such as growing the risk of high cholesterol and type 2 diabetes. The combination of high blood pressure, diabetes, and poor cholesterol will significantly raise the risk of cardiac attacks. Following a balanced diet can be very effective in addressing this problem.

Several foods and beverages, as you can see, will raise your blood pressure, mostly from hidden salt. Eating a ton of salt is possible without being conscious of it, just make sure you scan the diet labeling where you can. When you have hypertension, restricting the consumption of sodium (maximum daily amount of 1500 mg), alcohol, caffeine, and fats are profoundly necessary. Speak to a health care professional regarding referring you to a nutritionist who will help you discover healthier choices and advice on cooking if that is a problem for you.

3.3 Daily Meal Plans for Controlling High Blood Pressure

There are some common plans which are useful and very helpful in the daily meal plans to control high blood pressure

DASH Diet

The DASH diet emphasizes the correct portion amounts, nutritional diversity, and nutrients. Find out how DASH will boost overall health and drive down overall blood pressure.

DASH stands for "Dietary Approaches to Stop Hypertension." DASH diet is a lifestyle guide to balanced eating intended to either control high blood pressure (hypertension) or avoid them. The DASH diet program was established in research sponsored by the National Institutes of Health to reduce the blood pressure without medication.

The DASH diet allows you to reduce your daily salt and consume a range of nutrient-rich foods that can lower blood pressure, such as potassium, magnesium, and calcium.

You could be able to lower the blood pressure by a few points in just two weeks while adopting the DASH diet. With time, the blood pressure (systolic blood pressure) can decrease by eight to 14 points, which may make a big difference to your health risks.

Since the DASH diet is a safe way to consume, it provides nutritional advantages in addition to merely reducing blood pressure. The DASH plan frequently supports the nutritional guidelines for the treatment of osteoporosis, obesity, cardiac failure, stroke, and diabetes.

DASH Diet: Sodium levels

The DASH diet promotes herbs, citrus, and low-fat dairy products and small quantities of whole grains, meats, seafood, and nuts.

There is also a reduced salt variant of the menu in comparison to the regular DASH formula. You may pick the diet edition to match your health needs:

Standard DASH Diet

You can consume up to 2,300 milligrams (mg) of sodium a day.

Lower Sodium DASH Diet

You can consume up to 1,500 mg of sodium a day.

Both variations of the DASH plan strive to reduce the body's level of sodium relative to what you would receive in a standard diet, which may lead to 3,400 mg or more of sodium a day.

The regular DASH diet follows that maximum sodium consumption should be held to less than 2,300 mg a day.

The maximum limit of 1,500 mg of sodium a day for all ages. If you aren't sure which amount of sodium is appropriate for you, speak to the doctor.

DASH Diet: What to Eat

Both variations of the DASH diet contain plenty of whole foods, berries, vegetables, and meat items that are low in calories. The DASH diet also contains some seafood, poultry, and legumes and, a few days a week, supports a limited amount of nuts and seeds.

You should consume several tiny quantities of red meat, desserts, and fats. DASH diet includes small amounts of saturated fat, Trans fat, and total fat.

Here's a breakdown at the suggested portions of the 2,000-calorie-a-day DASH diet from the growing food category.

Grains: 6 to 8 Servings a Day

Grains include wheat, cereals, beans, and pasta. Examples of one-grain meal provide one slice of whole-wheat bread, 1 ounce of dried cereal, or 1/2 cup of cereal, beans, or pasta cooked.

Concentrate on whole grains because they provide more flavor and minerals than processed grains. For starters, instead of white rice, use brown rice, whole-wheat pasta instead of standard pasta, and whole-grain bread rather than white bread. Look for goods that are called "100 percent whole grain" or "100 percent whole wheat." Obviously, grains are low in calories. Hold them this way, stopping sauces of butter, milk, and cheese.

Vegetables: 4 to 5 Servings A Day

Tomatoes, cabbage, broccoli, sweet potatoes, greens, and other vegetables are filled with protein, calcium, and minerals such as potassium and magnesium. Examples of one serving provide 1 cup of fresh green leafy vegetables or 1/2 cup of fresh or cooked vegetables.

Don't only see vegetables as side dishes, a nutritious mix of vegetables served over brown rice or whole-wheat noodles will act as the main meal.

Both fresh and frozen vegetables are good options. Choose those that are branded as low sodium or without added salt while purchasing frozen and canned vegetables.

Be innovative to increase the number of servings you bring in each day. For example, reduce the amount of meat in half and double up on the vegetables in a stir-fry.

Fruits: 4 to 5 Servings A Day

To become a nutritious part of a meal or snack, several fruits require no planning. These are filled with fiber, potassium, and magnesium like carrots and are usually small in fat — coconuts are an exception.

Examples of a serving involve one small fruit, one-half cup of raw, frozen or canned fruit, or four ounces of water.

Take a slice of fruit with meals and one as a snack, and finish out the day with a new fruit treat served with a low-fat yogurt dollop.

Whenever necessary, set on edible peels. The peels of apples, pears, and other fruits give the recipes a fascinating texture and provide good nutrients and fiber.

Bear in mind that citrus fruits and juices, such as grapefruit, may interfere with other drugs, so consult with your doctor or pharmacist and see whether they're OK.

While picking canned fruit or juice, make sure there is no artificial sugar.

Dairy: 2 to 3 Servings A Day

Significant sources of calcium, vitamin D, and protein are meat, eggs, bacon, and other dairy foods. But the trick is to make sure you choose low-fat or fat-free dairy foods, since else they may be a big source of fat because most of them are unhealthy.

Examples of one serving include 1 skim cup of 1 percent milk, one low-fat cup yogurt, of 1 1/2 ounces of part-skim cheese.

Although providing a sweet treat, low-fat or fat-free frozen yogurt will help you increase the number of dairy products you consume. Add fruit for a wholesome twist.

When you have difficulty digesting dairy foods, select lactose-free items, or try taking an over-the-counter drug containing the lactase enzyme, which can mitigate or avoid the lactose sensitivity symptoms.

Go on standard and even fat-free cheeses comfortably, because they are normally high in sodium.

Healthy Beef, Poultry and Fish

Beef may be a good source of calcium, B vitamins, iron, and zinc for six one-ounce portions or less a day. Use lean varieties and try no more than six single-ounce portions a day. Cutting down on your portion of meat will allow more space for vegetables. Single serving sources involve one egg or 1 ounce of cooked beef, poultry, or fish. Trim the skin and fat away from beef and poultry and instead boil, broil, barbecue or roast instead of frying in butter. Eat nutritious seafood, e.g., trout, herring, and tuna. These fish species are rich in fatty omega-3 acids, which are safe for your skin.

Nuts, Seeds, and Legumes: 4 To 5 Servings A Week

Peanuts, sunflower seeds, kidney beans, peas, lentils, and other products are healthy sources of magnesium, potassium, and protein. These are also made of fiber and phytochemicals that can guard against many tumors and cardiovascular diseases. Serving sizes are small and are meant to be served just a few days a week as the calorie value of such items is higher. Definitions of one serving involve 1/3 cup almonds, two spoonful's of seeds or nut butter, or 1/2 cup of beans or peas.

Due to their fat content, nuts often get a poor name, but they contain good forms of fat — monounsaturated fat and omega-3 fatty acid. Nonetheless, nuts are rich in calories and enjoy them mildly. Attempt to add the stir-fries, salads, or cereals. Soya-based foods, such as tofu and tempeh, maybe a healthy substitute to meat as they contain all the amino acids that your body requires to create, much like beef, a full protein.

Fats and Oils: 2 To 3 Servings A Day

Fat lets the body digest essential minerals, which strengthens the immune system in your body. Yet the chance of heart failure, diabetes, and obesity is raised by too much weight.

The DASH diet focuses on healthy monounsaturated fats by restricting overall fat to fewer than 30 percent of daily calories from food. Sources with one serving provide one teaspoon with soft margarine, one tablespoon of mayonnaise, or two teaspoons of salad dressing.

The key dietary culprits are saturated fat and Trans fat in raising the chance of coronary heart disease. By restricting the use of beef, butter, dairy, whole milk, cream, and eggs in your diet, along with foods produced from lard, strong shortenings, and palm and coconut oils, DASH helps reduce your daily saturated fat to less than 6 percent of your total calories. Avoid trans-fat, typically present in packaged items such as crackers, baked goods, and fried products. Scan the margarine and salad dressing product labeling, and you can select products that are lowest in saturated fat and clear of Tran's fat.

Sweets: 5 Servings or Fewer a Week

When adopting the DASH diet, you don't have to banish desserts entirely. Just go gentle on them. Definitions of one serving include one spoonful of sugar, jelly or jam, 1/2 cup sorbet, or 1 cup lemonade. Choose those that are fat-free or low-fat while consuming desserts, such as sorbets, fruit ices, candies, hard candy, graham crackers, and low-fat cookies.

Sugar substitutes such as aspartame (NutraSweet, Equal) and sucralose (Splenda) can help to satisfy your sweet tooth while saving on sugar. Yet mind you do need to make good use of them. Swapping a diet cola with a normal cola is Fine, just not because of a more balanced liquid-like low-fat milk or just plain soda. Cut down on artificial sugar that has little intrinsic benefit but is capable of piling on calories.

Dash Diet: Alcohol and Caffeine

Too much alcohol will raise blood pressure. The Dietary Recommendations suggest that people restrict alcohol to no more than two beverages a day and that women reduce it to one or less.

The DASH diet is not for caffeine intake. It is uncertain whether caffeine affects blood pressure. But caffeine can trigger your blood pressure to rise momentarily, at least.

If you either have elevated blood pressure or suspect your blood pressure is impaired by caffeine, speak to the doctor about the intake of caffeine.

DASH Diet and Weight Loss

Although the DASH diet is not really a weight-loss plan, you can potentially shed excess pounds, and it will help direct you into making healthy decisions regarding food.

The DASH diet normally contains about 2,000 calories a day. When you are attempting to lose weight, you may require fewer calories to consume. You will still choose to change your serving targets according to your specific situation, something that the health care staff may help you determine.

Tips for Cutting Back On Sodium

The products that shape the basis of the DASH diet are, of course, low in sodium. Therefore, you're likely to reduce your sodium consumption by actually adopting the DASH plan. You can also eliminate sodium by use sodium-free spices or aromas in your food instead of salt. Not using salt while frying rice, pasta, or hot cereal. Rinsing canned products to avoid any of the sodium. Purchasing items called "no added salt," "sodium-free," "low sodium," or "really low sodium." One table salt tablespoon contains 2,325 mg of sodium. You may be shocked when you read food labeling on exactly how much sodium those packaged products produce.

Even low-fat soups, frozen peas, ready-to-eat cereals, and local deli-sliced turkey foods you may have thought healthy often produce tons of sodium. When selecting low-sodium foods and drinks, you may note a change in taste. If items are too boring, add in low-sodium products slowly and cut down on table salt before you hit your sodium target. That will allow you room to change your palate. The usage of salt-free seasoning mixes of herbs and spices may often help the process. It will take your taste buds many weeks to get accustomed to less salty products.

Putting the pieces of the DASH diet together

To get going on the DASH diet, follow these strategies:

Change Slowly

If you consume either one or maybe two servings of fruits or vegetables a day, consider incorporating one serving at lunch and one serving at dinner. Instead of going entirely to all whole grains, begin by having one or two of your whole grain servings. Gradually growing fruits, vegetables, and whole grains will also help avoid bloating or diarrhea that may happen if you are not accustomed to having a diet with plenty of fiber. You should also use items over the counter that help reduce the gas from beans and vegetables.

Reward Successes and Forgive Slip-Ups

Reward yourself for your successes with a non-food surprise; watch a video, purchase a book, and get together with a buddy. Particularly when learning anything fresh, everyone slips away. Notice the lifestyle shift is a long-term operation. Figure out what caused the failure, and then just take up the DASH diet where you left off.

Add a Physical Activity

Consider growing your physical exercise in addition to practicing the DASH plan to improve your blood pressure, reducing attempts even further. The use of both DASH eating and physical exercise allows it more probable that the blood pressure will be reduced.

Get support If You Need It

If you have difficulty holding on with your diet, speak to your doctor or nutritionist about it. You might be getting some ideas to help you adhere to the DASH plan.

Know, being good is not an all-or-nothing idea. Most notably, you consume healthy meals and lots of choice on average-both to keep your diet balanced and to prevent fatigue or extremes. And you can get all of these with the DASH diet.

Protein Diet

The Protein Diet is nothing drastic, but it is exceptionally balanced. Throughout over 100 trials conducted, the Diet and Exercise Protein plan was shown not only to encourage weight reduction but also to avoid and regulate many of the world's biggest killers, including diabetes, obesity, and cardiac failure.

The Protein Food Plan incorporates the current medical evidence to include the nutritional recommendations to help you prevent and even restore illnesses that will strip you of the better health you need to live a successful life.

A brief overview of the Protein Diet is provided below. Scroll down to the' Food Options for a Lifetime of Healthy Health ' segment for all the information.

"GO" Foods On The Protein Diet Include:

- Fruits
- Vegetables
- Whole Grains (like whole-wheat bread, brown rice, whole-wheat pasta, and oatmeal)
- Starchy Vegetables (like potatoes, corn, and yams)
- Legumes such as beans (like black beans, pinto beans, and garbanzo beans); peas; and lentils
- Lean Calcium-Rich Foods such as nonfat dairy milk, nonfat yogurt, and fortified soymilk
- Fish (a rich source of omega-3-fatty acids)
- Lean Sources of Protein (very low in saturated fat) such as skinless white poultry; lean red meat like bison and venison; and plant sources of protein, such as legumes and soy-based foods like tofu and edamame (soybeans)

"Caution" (less is better) Foods Include:

- Oils
- Refined Sweeteners such as sugar, corn syrup, and honey
- Salt

- Refined grains such as white bread, white pasta, and white rice

"Stop" (none is optimal) Foods Include:

- Saturated-Fat-Rich Foods such as butter; tropical oils like coconut oil; fatty meats; and dairy foods like cheese, cream, and whole/low-fat milk
- Organ Meats
- Processed Meats such as hot dogs, bacon, and bologna
- Partially Hydrogenated Vegetable Oils
- Cholesterol-Rich Foods like egg yolks

Unrefined Complex Carbohydrates

Five or more regular intakes of whole grains (such as maize, spinach, rye, brown rice, barley, quinoa, and millet); starchy vegetables (such as carrots, yams, and winter squash); chestnuts; and legumes (beans, peas, and lentils). A portion is ½ cup cooked. For whole-grain bread items (such as pieces of bread, bagels, and crackers), one serving is one ounce, which is normally half a typical serving.

Restricted as much as possible processed grains (such as white bread, white rice, and white pasta). Yet note that "white" doesn't automatically mean "unhealthy." There are a number of healthy white products, such as cauliflower, white potatoes, jicama, and non-fat yogurt.

Vegetables

5 Servings (preferably more) regular. A serving shall be 1 cup raw or 1/2 cup cooked. Experience a number of shades, from dark green, black, red, and white. The more vegetables, and other low-calorie-dense foods you consume, the less calorie counting is required. You're just going to consume fewer calories normally and lose bodyweight.

Fruit

Three or more parts every day of entire fruits. A serving fits into your hand on most fruits. Examples cover both fresh and dried fruits, including fruits that are frozen, including canned without added sugar. Enjoy fruit as a whole, not fruit juices. And don't trust dumb science, which says that fruit is fattening. Quite the reverse! People lose 100 pounds, and more, on the fruit-rich diet of Protein.

Dairy and/or Dairy Substitutes

2 Regular portions of dairy food and/or dairy substitutes.

Choose among nonfat milk (1 cup), nonfat yogurt (3/4 cup), and nonfat ricotta and cottage cheese variants (1/2 cup) for dairy products. Use simple non-fat milk, not aromatized variants such as cocoa. There is also an appropriate Nonfat Lactaid.

For dairy milk alternatives, select those that strongly suit calcium, vitamins D and B-12, and protein to the nutritional abundance of nonfat cow's milk. Optimal options tend to be (original or unsweetened) fortified soymilks. In fact, almond and rice milk perform high for calcium, D, and B-12, but negatively for protein. So if you're consuming a cup of almond or rice milk, add a light, protein-rich food like 1/2 cup of cooked legumes (beans) or two egg whites to your normal diet. Steer clear of milk from the coconut, since it includes saturated fat.

Assure whether they have very few to no added sugars, salt, and saturated fat for all fresh milk replacements.

Note: Most plant foods are high in calcium content, such as leafy greens such as collard greens, turnip greens and kale, and tofu and tempeh.

Protein-Rich Animal Foods

Like fish, white poultry, lean meat

Eating no more than one servings a day. One serving is cooked about $3\frac{1}{2}$ to 4 ounces (the equivalent of a card deck).

Below are "Strong" to "Bad" fish/poultry/meat options graded as:

Best: Omega-3-rich species (like tuna, sardines, herring, mackerel, and trout); Choose from at least twice a week. Pick types that are very-low-sodium or no-salt-added, whether you are using frozen seafood, such as canned sardines.

Good: Most other fish, plus shelled mollusks (clams, oysters, mussels, scallops).

Satisfactory: Crustaceans (shrimp, crab, lobster),

 Poultry (white meat, skinless),

 Game meat (bison, venison, elk), optimally free-range, and grass-fed.

Poor: Red meat (beef, pork, veal, lamb, goat). For all red meat choices, select cuts that are under 30% fat.

Restrict "Satisfying" options to no more than 1 serving a week and "Poor" options to no more than 1 serving a month for better heart-healthy results.

Egg's Whites

Up to 2 a day. When you prefer egg whites to other terrestrial animal foods such as white poultry and lean beef, you can consume more. The nutrition equivalent of one serving of poultry or meat is around seven egg whites. Steer clear of egg yolks, including excessive cholesterol in the diet.

Protein-Rich Plant Foods:

Legumes like beans, peas, and lentils

Soy products like tofu and edamame

For optimum cholesterol reduction and the greatest opportunity to reverse atherosclerosis (heart disease), use plant foods such as beans on most days instead of soil-based animal feed such as poultry and beef. And indeed, a plant-based diet will help you get enough protein.

If You Want To Lose Weight

Go crazy on vegetables. The stronger the most vegetables like dark green, red, orange, yellow vegetables! They are also the safest weight reduction products.

Restrict dense-calorie products such as dried grains (pieces of bread, crackers, frozen cereals), dried fruits, nuts, and seeds. Remove condensed or processed sweeteners. They are both packing a ton of calories into very limited quantities of food. If you concentrate on high-water, high-fiber foods like cooked grains (such as oatmeal and brown rice), beans, and whole fruits, you'll find it far simpler to stay full and comfortable and reduce hunger. Such products are low in the number of calories. You are supposed to eat better-then weigh less.

Steer clear of juices for fruit and vegetables because they have less satiety than whole fruits and vegetables.

If Your Weight Is Fine

Let's toast! Eat as many whole grains, potatoes, legumes (like beans and peas) as you like, and fruits. Eat more calorie-dense products like avocados and nuts but hold them under balance to maintain your weight. Reduce the consumption of avocados to no more than 2 ounces a day. Restricted to no more than 1 ounce a day walnuts, flaxseeds, almonds, pumpkin seeds, pecans, pistachios, sunflower seeds, filberts (hazelnuts), peanuts, cashews, and macadamia nuts.

Caution (the less, the better)

While foods that are not recommended for "caution," this list offers direction even when food options are restricted.

Refined Fats & Oils

Limit ALL oils intake to not even more than one teaspoon per 1000 calories eaten, particularly if you are attempting to lose weight since the oils have the highest calorie density of any product or ingredient.

Refined or Concentrated Sweeteners

A proposed thumb rule among healthier people who want to use sweeteners is a limit of 2 teaspoons of fruit juice concentrated or one tablespoon of other artificial sweeteners (such as barley malt, corn, or rice syrup) for every 1000 calories ingested. None are optimal. Avoid sugar with fructose and high fructose maize.

Salt and High-Sodium Foods and Condiments

Stop incorporating salt, and products heavily salted, pickled and roasted. Limit foods with more than 1 mg of sodium per calorie such that, based on age, no more than 1200 to 1500 mg of sodium per day.

It's one of the most effective stuff for reducing blood pressure you might do.

Refined Grains

Restrict products with processed grains (such as white noodles, white bread, and white rice) as far as possible.

Stop (think about it first)

Facing foods in the "Stop" category, check for "Go" options, and "Caution" foods where appropriate. "Avoid" products will substantially weaken your personal health priorities despite their high concentration of saturated oil, hydrogenated fat, cholesterol, and/or sodium. Be cautious about headline-grabbing media reports, which indicate otherwise. Unfortunately, the traditional diet comprises primarily of items labeled "Caution" and "Stop."

Animal Fats, Tropical Oils, and Processed Refined Oils

These involve butter, coconut oil, palm kernel oil, lard, chicken fat, palm sugar, peanut butter, chocolate, margarine, hydrogenated and partially hydrogenated vegetable oils, and shortening.

Meats

Such as fatty meats, organ meats, and processed meats (hot dogs, bacon, and bologna).

Whole and Low-Fat Dairy

All cheese, cream, cream cheese, half-and-half, ice cream, milk, sour cream, and yogurt, unless fat-free and low in sodium like.

- **Nuts**
- Coconuts
- **Salt Substitutes**
- Potassium chloride
- **Miscellaneous**
- Egg yolks
- Deep-fried foods
- Non-dairy whipped toppings
- Rich desserts and pastries
- Salty snack foods

Heart-Healthy Diet
What are the benefits of heart-healthy eating?
It's crucial to consume a good healthy diet to control your blood pressure and decrease the risk of heart disease, stroke, and any other health risks.
Get Quality Nutrition from Healthy Food Sources
Aim to eat a diet that's rich in:

- Fruits
- Vegetables
- Whole-grains
- Low-fat dairy products
- Skinless poultry and fish
- Nuts and legumes
- Non-tropical vegetable oils

Limit

- Saturated and trans fats
- Sodium
- Red meat (if you do eat red meat, compare labels and select the leanest cuts available)
- Sweets and sugar-sweetened beverages

Be sure to collaborate in your home with the "chefs" to prepare for any nutritional adjustments that could be made together. Seek the heart-healthy dishes while eating at home. Check for safe choices while eating outdoors.
Read the Labels
You may select products more effectively by making a habit of consulting food labeling. Search for products containing saturated fat or trans-fat causes that will raise cholesterol. Eating foods rich in sodium (salt) will raise blood pressure. The greater the salt level, the greater the blood pressure would usually be.

Look For the Heart-Check Mark

With so many advertising campaigns in the grocery store being launched, it may be hard to learn what truly is safe. The Heart Associations had created the Heart-symbol to make things simpler. When you see this mark on food packages, it indicates the drug follows the saturated fat, Tran's fat and sodium requirements for a single portion of the nutritional commodity for healthy persons over age 2.

Healthy Snacks to Eat With High Blood Pressure

High blood pressure worries us, mainly because it's too normal. About one in three adults would suffer a period of high blood pressure. But that doesn't imply you will also suffer from it. A big part of high blood pressure fending off stems from what you consume. If you're searching for a late-night or midday snack, here's what you can pick.

Carrots and Hummus

Hummus is a tasty snack when combined with chips. But because tortilla chips also have a high salt level, switch them out for carrots without losing your health to get a sincere snap. Carrots are filled with vitamin A and antioxidants, which are beneficial to the skin. Hummus is a low-sodium dip but sticks on one serving.

Greek Yogurt with Berries

Grab a Greek vanilla yogurt (Greek yogurt has a low sugar content than normal yogurt) for a satisfying snack and mix it with fresh berries. Berries include phytonutrients, which help to keep your heart healthy. Plus, they're filled with fiber that's healthy for the heart as well and leaves you feeling full.

Apple Slices and Peanut Butter

We often see peanut butter as bad, but it's perfect for you in moderation, and it's also tasty. It includes calcium, plus heart-healthy fats, rendering it the ultimate snack add-on. On the other side, apples may minimize inflammation in the walls of the artery, as well as minimize cholesterol. In certain respects, they're perfect for the heart, and having a little touch of peanut butter just makes us stronger.

Whole Wheat Crackers with Tuna

The one thing to test while buying whole wheat crackers is their low sodium quality. A reduced-sodium diet is known to be no less than 140 milligrams per meal. Crackers are often flavored with salt to enhance flavor. Yet combine low-sodium crackers for a protein-packed snack with a helping of canned tuna that will hold you fresh. The complex carbohydrates break down in the bloodstream more gradually, thereby avoiding an unnecessary increase of blood sugar.

Dark Chocolate Covered Bananas

When you want a tasty treat, you might need to top you up with more than one ounce of dark chocolate. Alternatively, bake pieces of banana filled in chocolate to make-ahead. They're chocolate sweet also contain heart-healthy banana vitamins and minerals like potassium. Potassium continuously prevents the heart from pumping and can overcome so much sodium.

Avoid salty snacks, such as chips and salsa, salted nuts, etc.

While knowing which snacks to consume, it's essential to also know which snacks to stop. Every type of jarred sauce, like salsa, also has a strong sodium content to enhance spice. Homemade salsa with whole-grain crackers is a nutritious snack, but one to resist is jarred salsa mixed with spicy tortilla chips. Nuts are indeed healthy for the core, so make sure to purchase the unsalted variety. For the body to work correctly, sodium is essential, so you just need around 500 milligrams a day. The Americans eat 3,400 milligrams a day on average. Too much sodium is a significant source of hypertension.

Chapter 4: Relationship between Blood Pressure and Weight Loss

Maintaining a proper weight has numerous advantages for the body. If you are overweight, it can help to reduce your blood pressure by reducing as little as five to 10 pounds.

A Few Great and Common Reasons To Manage Your Weight

Overweight puts you at a higher risk of having health conditions. A modest weight reduction will offer substantial health benefits. Are you conscious that you can receive health benefits by losing as little as 10 pounds? For specific overweight individuals (those with a body mass index (BMI) of 25 or greater), only a modest weight reduction may help to control or reduce high blood pressure.

Weight reduction decreases cardiac pressure. Getting overweight places an additional burden on the back, raising the risk of developing high blood pressure and harm to your blood vessels, which can contribute to severe threats to your health.

Overweight is a disorder that is rapidly common all over the world. The latest figures, which are presumably optimistic, indicate that at least 500 000 000 individuals globally are overweight as characterized by a body mass index (BMI) between 25.0 and 29.9, and an estimated 250 000 000 are obese with a BMI of 30.0 or higher. Current statistics suggest that as many as 66% of the adult population is obese or overweight.

Overweight and obesity are contributing factors known for cardiovascular disease (CVD), stroke, noninsulin-dependent diabetes (NIDDM), many cancers, and many other diseases. Hypertension is also a contributing factor.

The association between overweight or obese and blood pressure and risk of hypertension is positive. A strong correlation between body weight and blood pressure was observed in people as early as the 1920s. Epidemiological trials have regularly verified this relationship in the intervening years. The study showed that hypertension is nearly twice as common in obese than both sexes, no obese. It is also observed that the risk ratio of 2.42 for younger people and 1.54 for older individuals for obese hypertension compared to no obese (BMI of less than 25). The Nurses Health Survey contrasted people with BMIs of less than 22 to those over 29 and observed a 2-to 6-fold hypertension rate in the obese.

4.1 Effects of Weight on Hypertension

As your body weight increases, it may increase your blood pressure. In reality, being obese can makes you more likely to acquire high blood pressure than when you're at your desirable body mass. About 70 percent of adults are overweight. By losing weight, you may reduce your chances of high blood pressure. Even small sums of weight loss can make a significant difference in preventing high blood pressure and treat it.

To see improvements in your blood pressure and general health, you don't have to sign on to a strenuous diet plan or dump a large amount of Weight. Before that happens, you start receiving health payoffs.

The scale doesn't even involve three of the most excellent perks.

Your Heart, And Your Life, Improve

The most significant gains are related more to a lower risk of stroke and heart attack. The benefits far outweigh your heart. Even a slight loss of Weight means more considerable energy and the capacity to do more activities. Plus, you'll boost your confidence and overall quality of life when you can do more.

(Almost) Instant Gratification

Your heart is strained by being overweight, which can lead to a host of health problems, including heart disease. You don't have to take 50 pounds off to see a progression. Losing as little as just 10 pounds can lower your blood pressure and start reducing your stress.

Better Numbers in 30 Days

Looking at what you eat will have the most significant influence on your blood pressure; however, exercise seems to be an essential component of success. Exercising can reduce blood pressure by much more than five to seven points. And just one month after increasing your activity you can see those results. A researcher says they aim for 30 minutes of exercise a day. Low-intensity exercises like walk and swim are simple ways to start a routine and begin to see promising changes on visits to your doctors.

How to Lose For Good

It takes hard work to stay on track, and it is worth the effort. It's the best way to retain the health benefits you'll gain from dropping a few pounds.

Use These Few Tips to Help You Keep Your Weight-Loss Plan Going

- Give a try to the DASH diet

(The plan was developed without medication to help lower blood pressure but is now an absolute favorite for anyone who needs to lose weight. "Think of less packaged food, less sodium, and many more vegetables and fruits." High fiber and less fat and sodium are also emphasized).

- Set specific and realistic goals. Start with 30 minutes on feet, three days a week.

- Get your team along. Build your network for support. Discuss your goals with your friends, family, and doctors and let them understand how they can improve. Get them to cheer you on board, and encourage you.
- Keep a log of exercise and diet for motivation and track what works and what doesn't.
- Grateful for your success. Feel free to reward yourself. Create a list of realistic "treats" even after the initial weight loss goal when you hit milestones. Did that keep it off for a month? Six months? Take a show, get a massage, or pick some other treat that will make you feel special.

4.2 Increasing Activities to Lower Blood Pressure and weight loss

Exercise Helps Manage Blood Pressure and Weight

Not only does physical activity help control high blood pressure (HBP or hypertension), but it also assists with weight management, cardiovascular strength, and stress. All good for your blood pressure is a good weight, a healthy heart, and emotional health in general.

Being Inactive Is Bad For Your Health

People who are not physically active have a high rate of health problems, like heart attack and stroke.

Finding the Time and Energy to Be More Active

Just get moving when it comes to physical activity. Find ways to enjoy the benefits and enjoy them as you progressively increase your level of activity.

Don't Be Afraid To Get Active

If you haven't been active for quite a while or if you are beginning a new workout or fitness plan, slowly take it. If you have heart disease or any other pre-existing condition, consult with your healthcare professional. It is best to start with something you enjoy slowly, like walking or riding a bicycle. Scientific proof indicates strongly that physical exercise is safe for nearly everyone. Besides, physical activity's health benefits far outweigh the risks.

Find Something You Like

Combine that with running if you appreciate the outdoors, and admire the nature as you jog or walk. If you are listening to audiobooks, please enjoy them by using an elliptical trainer.

Such practices are particularly beneficial if performed regularly:

- Walking, hiking or stair-climbing
- Running, jogging, bicycling, swimming or rowing
- Fitness programs
- Some activities including team sports, a dance class or fitness games

Mix It Up! Adding Variety to Your Workout Is Right for You

Staying engaged and inspired is supported by a variety of activities. When you have targets of strength and endurance (using weights, resistance bands, yoga, and stretching exercises), you can help lower the risk of injuries, and you can sustain a high degree of heart-healthy fitness for several years.

Know What Moderate Means For You

If you're hurting yourself right from the start, you're less likely to proceed. Concentrate on doing something which will raise the heart rate to a healthy level. If you are consistently physically involved for more extended stretches or at a higher strength, you are going to gain more. You don't exaggerate. Too much exercise will give you muscles that are weak and raise the chance of injury.

Make It Social

Try walking with your neighbor, friend, or partner. Taking a chance to work out. You should keep yourself focused and inspired to move forward.

Look forward to something that suits the goals:

- Pay yourself. (Set aside a little money for each workout. For one month, spend your money into something that inspires you to start performing hard, like new songs to listen while exercising or a new exercise).

- Celebrate your milestones. (Fitness is a daily part of your life, so it is essential to find ways to taste your success. Report on your walk or run and write a congratulatory note as you hit a landmark, or relax every 100 miles, any motivation you should keep going regularly).

Warm-Up and Cool Down

Warming up and cooling down afterward allows the heart to move slowly back and forth from rest to activity. You often reduce the chance of injuries or soreness.

Your warm-up will take at least 10 minutes longer if you're older or long inactive.

Time to cool down is also particularly important. You can dramatically decrease blood pressure, which can be harmful and cause muscle cramping if you avoid exercising too fast.

In addition to the workout, certain soothing yoga poses will also increase versatility.

Practice Breath Control

Make sure you consistently breathe during the warm-up, workout, and refreshment. Holding your breath will increase blood pressure and cause muscle tightness. Deep breathing will also help you to relax regularly.

Need To Consult The Doctor Before Increasing The Activity Level?

Healthy people do not typically have to contact a healthcare provider until they become physically active. People with medical illnesses should speak to their health care providers to find out if their diseases hinder their ability to exercise regularly.

How to Calculate Heart Rate?

In order to measure your heart rate goal, you need to know your heart rate at rest. Resting your heart rate is the number of times your heart beats at rest per minute. After a full night's sleep and until you get out of bed, the perfect time to check your heart rate. In general, the heart rate of a person is 60-100 beats per minute. However, it is usually lower for people who are genuinely fit. In addition, a restful heart rate often increases with age.

The best spots to find your heartbeat are the wrists within your forearm, neck side, or foot top. Place your finger on your pulse, and check the number of pulses in 60 seconds to get the most accurate measurement.

How Much To Exert Yourself?

When you know your heart rate at rest, you can calculate your heart rate goal. Target cardiac levels allow you to assess your initial fitness level and track your fitness program progress. You do this by consistently checking your pulse when exercising and remaining within 50-85% of your heart rate. This range is referred to as your heart rate goal.

Remember, the Pacing Is Important

It is important to keep pace when exercising. If you just start a plan, target the lower part of your goal zone in the first few weeks (50 percent). Step up to the top of the goal zone (85 percent). You will exercise safely at up to 85% of your average heart rate after six months or more of daily exercise. But you don't have to work out to stay in shape.

Using Fitness Trackers and Health Apps for Heart Health

Health applications and portable fitness bands will allow you to set realistic goals and targets. This is also very inspiring to see how you are progressing.

A Note about Hot Tubs and Saunas

High blood pressure individuals should be able to handle both saunas and their blood pressure. Consult your health care provider for advice if you have elevated blood pressure and have questions about hot tubes and Saunas. The heat from hot tubs and saunas is contributing to the expansion of blood vessels (called vasodilation). Even during regular activities, vasodilation takes place as a short walk.

If your doctor advised you to stop light exercise, you could also suggest hot tubs and saunas. Persons with high blood pressure must not switch between cold water and hot tubes or saunas because this may cause blood pressure to rise. Alcohol and the use of a sauna are also not a healthy idea, so don't put them together.

4.3 Obesity and Hypertension

Both hypertension and Weight must be managed to be healthy; obesity and hypertension are major health problems.

The Incidence of Hypertension and Obesity

One prominent study reported that excessive body weight (including overweight and obesity) accounted for around 26% of men's and 28% of females ' hypertension, and about 23% of men's and 15% of women's coronary cardiac diseases.

Obesity individuals have a rise in fat tissues that increases their vascular resistance and thus increases the function that the heart does to pump blood throughout the body.

What Is Obesity?

Obesity is a health condition that has developed by excess body fat to the point that it can affect health.

Obesity is also defined as a condition of abnormal or excessive fat accumulation in adipose tissue, to the extent that health is impaired.

The definition of obesity varies according to what one would be reading. Overweight and obesity, in general, indicate a weight more significant than that, which is a healthy weight requirement for a person. For the storage of energy, heat insulation, shock absorption, and other functions, a certain amount of body fat required.

Body mass index (BMI) defines obesity at its best. The height and weight of one person determine his or her measure of body weight. The body mass index (BMI) is equal to a person's weight in kilograms (kg) divided into meters (M) measured by their height. BMI Ex body weight relative to height, and Adults have a strong correlation with total body caloric density.

For Example, An adult with a BMI of 25-29.9 is overweight, and an adult with a BMI higher than 30 is obese. A person with an 18.5-24.9 BMI shall have a healthy weight. A person is morbidly obese if his or her BMI is over 40.

What Is Hypertension?

Hypertension (high blood pressure) refers to blood pressure on the inner walls of the arteries. The high blood pressure diagnosis cannot be made if the patient is diseased or is already taking medications for blood pressure.

High blood pressure is dependent on the average of two or more accurately calculated measurements of the blood pressure after the initial test for any one of two or more visits.

Doctors use the classifications mention below:

Normal Blood Pressure

Systolic: equal to or less than 120 mmHg, and diastolic pressure: equals to or less than around 80 mmHg

Pre-Hypertension

Systolic pressure: 120-139 mmHg or diastolic pressure: 80-89 mmHg

Hypertension

- In Stage 1: systolic: 140-159 mmHg or diastolic: 90-99 mmHg
- In Stage 2: systolic will be greater than or equal to 160 mmHg or diastolic will be greater than or equal 100 mmHg

Types of Hypertension

There are two forms of hypertension: primary and secondary hypertension. Most individuals with high blood pressure have essential high blood pressure.

Essential hypertension is not well known and can be induced by a variety of causes like history, kidney complications (due to hypoxia, pharmaceuticals, dietary deficiency, obesity, infection, genetic factors) and neural operation.

Secondary hypertension is less prevalent due to another underlying medical condition, such as kidney disease, oral contraceptives, pheochromocytoma, primary hyperaldosteronism, Cushing syndrome, and aorta coarctation.

Treating Hypertension

Blood pressure (antihypertensives) medications should be used for people with hypertension. Those with high blood pressure medication need to remember that everyone reacts differently to these drugs and that two or three medicines may be required to maintain healthy blood pressure.

Blood pressure medicines will taper or stop if weight loss occurs, and normal blood pressure is reached. No medical trials revealed that those medicines for blood pressure perform better or are healthier in obese patients.

Many forms of drugs may be used, and physicians can think about the dangers and benefits of the available options.

Possible solutions are:

- ACE inhibitors
- Low dose diuretics
- Calcium channel blocker

The low-dose thiazide drug is less expensive and will have little to no effect on the absorption of glucose to lipids, which may be a concern with the other antihypertensive medicines.

Knowing Your Risk for Hypertension

Obesity, abdominal obesity, and weight gain are measures of the risk of hypertension. Obesity is measured by the Weight and height of a body mass index (BMI). In most cultures, BMI is strongly associated with direct measurements of body fat. Average BMI is 20-25, 25-29.9 overweight, and more than 30 obesity. BMI is not only important for assessing the risk of hypertension, but also for fat distribution.

Abdominal obesity is considered a fat collection in the abdominal region. The waist circumference is more significant than 102 cm (40 in) in men and 88 cm (35 in) in women. Abdominal obesity has the most significant impact on how anyone has high blood pressure. Weight gain was linked to an increased risk of hypertension development.

For women who added 10-22 pounds and for women who gained more than 55 pounds, the relative risks were 1.7 and 5.2. In other words, women who weighed over 55 pounds were three times more likely than women who weighed less Weight. Weight loss, on the other hand, may lead to a significant decrease in blood pressure. A research found that a 10 percent weight loss in a four-year follow-up of 181 hypertensive overweight patients caused an average 4.3/3.8 mmHg drop in blood pressure. Obesity patients have other significant health risks, and abdominal obesity patients are at the highest risk. Heart disorders risk increase if a person has excess abdominal fat, elevated blood pressure, high blood cholesterol levels, heart disease, a clear family history of heart disease, or a male is obese before age 40, Heart disease risk increases. Fat distribution and overall bodyweight appear to be related to the defects of lipid and glucose metabolism, which is why patients with obesity have a higher risk of diabetes mellitus.

Obesity raises the risk of heart disease by increasing levels of LDL cholesterol (bad cholesterol) and reducing HDL-cholesterol (good cholesterol). This causes atherosclerosis (heart artery hardening) that can lead to a heart attack.

Obesity also raises the chances of diabetes by reducing the immunity to glucose and predisposing to left-ventricular hypertrophy production (cardiac expansion). For patients with obesity, left ventricular hypertrophy is likely because the heart is forced to pump blood more intensely across the body. Each pound of fat, according to some figures, takes roughly a mile more blood vessels to provide oxygen and nutrients.

Did You Know?

Obesity and hypertension are closely related (high blood pressure). Hypertension is the most common explanation for visits to their physicians by non-pregnant adults and prescription drugs, and obesity is the most common cause of high blood pressure.

The number of obese people is rising every day. Specific medical conditions linked to obesity include reduced life expectancy, cardiovascular disease, diabetes mellitus, gallstones, arthritis, elevated cholesterol (blood lipids), stroke, sleep apnea, and cancer (male colon and prostate, female uterine and gallbladder cancers).

What to Remember With Hypertension and Obesity

The essential thing to note is that obesity is connected to high blood pressure, and hypertension is linked to many other diseases that affect overall health and lifespan.

Medications against hypertension must be started if hypertension is confirmed. However, due to weight loss, a substantial drop in blood pressure could cause the number of drugs taken to be decreased, or the number of medications considered to be reduced. Prevention is safer than any other treatment.

Carry some lifestyle improvements in the form of weight loss (maintaining BMI 18.5 to 24.9kg/m2), DASH diet (eating fruit, vegetables, and low-fat milk products with decreased saturated and total fat content), sodium decrease in the diet (sodium 2.4g, sodium 6g), increased physical activity (30 minutes a day) and mild alcohol consumption. Weight loss is the first step in lowering high blood pressure and enhancing the quality of life.

4.4 Maintaining Weight for a Life Time

Unfortunately, even people that lose Weight ultimately get back to it. However, just about 20 percent of dieters who become overweight lose Weight and hold it away over the long term.

Yet don't let that stop you. There are a variety of clinically validated ways to hold the Weight off, including stress management.

These techniques can be just what you need to offer your advantages to the statistics and maintain your weight loss.

Why People Regain Weight

There are several common explanations for why people regain their Weight. Most of them are due to unreasonable aspirations and feelings of hardship.

Restrictive Diets

Heavy calories can slow down your metabolism and change your appetite control hormones, both of which lead to weight recovery.

Wrong Mindset

If you find a diet a rapid fix instead of a long-term approach to improving your fitness, you're more likely to quit and lose your lost Weight.

Lack of Sustainable Habits

Several diets are based on willpower other than habits you can incorporate into your daily life. They focus on rules instead of lifestyle changes, which may discourage you and prevent weight maintenance.

Exercise Often

Regular exercise plays a significant role in controlling weight. This could allow you to burn out more calories and increase your metabolism, two things important to maintain energy balance. When you have an energy balance, it ensures that you eat the same number of calories. Your Weight is also more likely to remain the same.

Many studies have shown that people who do moderate physical exercise at least 200 minutes a week (30 minutes a day) following weight loss are more likely to retain their Weight. For some instances, much higher levels of physical work may be required to maintain weight effectively. One study found that one hour of exercise a day is suitable for those who want to avoid weight loss.

It is important to remember that weight loss exercise is most effective when done in combination with other improvements in lifestyles, maintaining a balanced diet. Exercise for at least thirty minutes each day will help to reduce your calories and burned calories.

Try Eating Breakfast Every Day

Eating breakfast will help you achieve your maintenance objectives. Breakfast eaters tend to have more balanced habits, such as more exercise and more fiber and micronutrients.

Breakfast is even one of the most common habits reported by people who maintain weight loss. One research found that 78% of 2 959 people who had a weight loss of 30 pounds (14 kg) for at least one year reported eating breakfast daily. Although people who eat breakfast tend to be very good at sustaining weight loss, there is a mixture of facts.

Research does not indicate that breakfast skipping necessarily results in weight gain or unhealthy eating habits. Indeed, missing breakfast can also help certain people experience weight loss and weight maintenance objectives. This may be one of the things the person gets down to. When you believe that breakfast eating allows you to achieve your goals, you should probably eat it. However, if you don't like breakfast or if you don't feel hungry in the morning, there's no harm to miss. People who eat breakfast tend to overall have healthy habits that can help them stay weighty. Skipping breakfast does not contribute to weight gain immediately.

Eat Lots of Protein

Eating plenty of protein will help you maintain your Weight because protein will help suppress appetite and encourage completeness. Protein raises body levels of certain hormones, which induce satiety and are important for the control of Weight. Protein has also been shown to reduce hormone levels that increase hunger. Protein effects on hormones and fullness will naturally reduce your daily calories, which is a significant factor in weight maintenance. In addition, protein takes considerable energy to break down the body.

Therefore, daily consumption will increase the amount of calories you burn throughout the day.

Based on many studies, protein effects on metabolism and appetite tend to be the most pronounced when approximately 30% of calories are absorbed by protein. In a 2000 calorie diet, that is 150 grams of protein.

Protein can benefit from encouraging completeness, increasing metabolism, and significantly reducing calorie intake.

Weigh Yourself Regularly

Monitoring your Weight by frequently stepping onto the scale can be an excellent way to control Weight. It is because it will remind you of your success and encourage weight management behavior. People that weigh themselves will also eat fewer calories all day long, which helps to sustain weight loss. For one study, people with a weight of six days a week ate an average of 300 fewer calories a day than people with less weight control.

How many times you weigh yourself is your personal preference. Others consider it beneficial to weigh on a regular basis while others test their Weight once a week or twice a week more effectively. Self-weighing can help control weight by keeping you informed of your success and behavior.

Be Mindful Of Your Carb Intake

Weight management will be easier to do if the types and quantities of carbohydrates you consume are taken into account. Too many processed carbohydrates, including white bread, white pasta, and fruit juices, can be hazardous to the maintenance of your Weight.

Such foods have been separated from their natural fiber to encourage their fullness. Fiber-low diets are related to weight gain and obesity. You will also reduce your net carb consumption by maintaining your weight loss. Several studies have shown that in some cases, Weight is more likely to be retained long-term by those adopting low-carb diets after weight loss.

Therefore, people who adopt low-carb diets eat fewer calories than they consume, which is required to maintain weight. It can help prevent weight recovery by reducing your intake of carbs, in particular those which are processed.

Lift Weights

A common side effect of weight loss is decreased muscle mass. This will limit your Weight because the lack of muscle reduces your metabolism, which ensures you eat fewer calories every day. Do any form of strength exercise, such as lifting weights, will help to prevent this muscle loss while preserving or even raising your metabolic rate?

Research suggests that people who lift Weight following weight loss are more likely to gain weight while retaining muscle mass. To benefit from these advantages, strength training is recommended at least twice a week. Your workout scheme will work for optimal results for all muscle groups. Lifting weights at minimum twice a week will help maintain weight by increasing your muscle mass, which is vital to keep a healthy metabolism.

Be Prepared For Setbacks

Setbacks on the weight loss journey are unavoidable. Occasionally you give in to an unwanted desire or miss a practicing. The occasional slip-up, though, does not mean that you will throw your goals down. Just continue and make better choices. This will also help prepare for events in the future, which will complicate healthy eating, such as a coming holiday or vacation. You will possibly experience a reversal or two following weight loss. You will solve challenges if you prepare ahead and get on track immediately.

Stick To Your Plan for Whole Week (Even On Weekends)

A habit that sometimes leads to a recovery of Weight is healthy eating on weekdays and cheating on weekends. This attitude also contributes to fast food that can compensate for weight loss efforts. If you get used to it, you might regain more Weight than you first lost.

Alternatively, evidence suggests that people who follow a regular diet during the week are more prone to long-term weight loss. One study showed that, relative to people who had more flexibility on weekends, the weekly consistency made people almost twice as likely to maintain Weight within five pounds (2.2 kg) for a year. Proper management of Weight is easier to do when you stick to healthy eating habits over the entire week, even on weekends.

Stay Hydrated

For a few purposes, drinking water is good for weight maintenance.

It promotes completeness and can help you verify calorie intake if you drink a glass or two before dinner. In one study, people who drank water before consuming meals decreased calorie consumption by 13% compared to people who did not drink water.

In addition, the amount of calories you eat during the day has risen marginally by drinking water. Drinking water can regularly encourage completeness and improve your metabolism, both essential weight loss factors.

Get Enough Sleep

Having enough sleep impacts weight management dramatically.

Sleep deprivation, in addition, seems to be a significant risk factor for adult weight gain and can interfere with weight maintenance. This is because insufficient sleep contributes to higher ghrelin, known as the "hunger hormone," because it raises appetite.

In addition, poor sleepers appear to have lower levels of lepton, an appetite-regulating hormone.

Moreover, those who sleep for a short time are exhausted and less driven to exercise and make good food choices. Find a way to change your sleep patterns if you don't get enough. It is best for weight management and good health to sleep for at least seven hours a night. Sleeping for a reasonable period of time will help maintain Weight by regulating your energy levels and hormones.

Control Stress Levels

Stress management is an essential aspect of weight regulation. High-stress levels can also improve weight recovery by increasing the cortisol level, which is a hormone that responds to stress. Consistently higher cortisol is associated with higher levels of bowel fat, increased appetite, and decreased food intake.

Stress is also a common cause for impulsive eating, even though you don't get hungry when you eat. Luckily, you can do many things to combat tension, including exercise, yoga, and meditation.

To reduce your weight, it is important to regulate stress levels, as excess stress will increase your weight by increasing your appetite.

Find a Support System

It can be hard to meet the weight targets alone. One approach is to find a support group to keep you responsible and probably collaborate with you in your safe lifestyle.

Some studies have shown that following your goals can help you manage weight, especially if that individual is a friend or spouse with similar healthy habits. One research analyzed the health habits of over 3,000 people and found that the other individual is more likely to follow their example if they are interested in healthy activities, such as exercise. Engaging a partner in a healthy lifestyle may increase the likelihood of your loss of Weight.

Track Your Food Intake

Many who monitor their food consumption in a journal, online food tracker, or app will sustain their weight loss more quickly.

Food trackers are useful as they improve the knowledge of how much you consume because they also offer specific details on how many nutrients and calories you consume. In addition, you can record your workout with several food monitoring apps to ensure that you get the amount you need to keep your Weight. Logging your consumption of food regularly will help maintain your weight loss by showing you how many nutrients and calories you consume.

Eat Plenty of Vegetables

Several studies link the high consumption of vegetables with better control of Weight.

For example, the calories of vegetables are small. You can eat significant portions without weight gain while still consuming a lot of nutrients. In addition, vegetables are rich in fiber, which increases full feelings and can minimize the amount of calories you consume during the day automatically. For these benefits of weight management, a serving or two vegetables are to be eaten at every meal. Vegetables are fiber-rich and calorie-low. Both of these properties can aid in maintaining weight.

Be Consistent

Consistency is important to maintain weight. More than the on-and-off diet, which ends with a return to old habits, you better stick to your current balanced diet and lifestyle.

While introducing a new "way of life" at first can seem daunting, making healthy choices is secondary to them. Your healthy lifestyle is carefree, and you can keep your Weight much easier. Maintaining weight loss is easy if you follow your new healthy habits instead of going back to your old way of life.

Practice Mindful Eating

Mindful eating is the activity of reacting to internal appetite signals and paying complete attention during the food cycle. It involves slowly eating without distractions and thoroughly chewing the food so you can feel the scent and flavor of your meal. If you eat that way, when you are entirely finished, you are more likely to stop feeding. If you feed when disturbed, it can be challenging to understand fullness. Studies have found that mindful eating helps to Reduce Weight by concentrating on habits typically associated with gaining weight, such as emotional intake. Therefore, those who eat attentively can keep their Weight without calorie counting. Careful eating is effective in managing weight as it helps you accept fullness and can discourage unsanitary habits, which typically contribute to weight gain.

Make Sustainable Changes to Your Lifestyle

The reason many people struggle to control their weight is that they are adopting unhealthy, long-term diets. Many end up feeling deprived, which also results in a higher weight gain than they have gained once they return to eating healthy. Maintaining weight loss requires healthy lifestyle changes. It is different for everybody, but ultimately it doesn't mean that we are too conservative, consistent, and making the right decisions as much as possible. It is better to avoid weight loss by adopting a healthy lifestyle than to obey the unrealistic restrictions that other weight-loss diets focus on. Diets may be restrictive and impractical, often leading to a reduction of Weight. Nonetheless, several quick improvements will help you stick to your routines and maintain your weight loss on a long term basis. You will learn during your journey that managing your weight is far more than what you eat. Exercise, rest, and mental health are also significant. Weight management is easy if you simply follow a healthy lifestyle instead of developing weight-loss diets.

4.5 Tips for Living with High Blood Pressure

Because hypertension does not typically cause any symptoms, you cannot worry about trying to cope. Nevertheless, treatment means you have to take anti-hypertensive medicines and make some adjustments in diet and lifestyle.

A significant risk factor in multiple illnesses, like heart attacks, strokes, and kidney failure, is high blood pressure. Therefore your body needs you to help prevent hypertension from causing more worry while you may feel well. You can also learn that controlling high blood pressure will put you at risk and provide emotional and social support.

Physical Activities

If you have high blood pressure, you need to keep your blood pressure stable to manage your blood pressure with some exercise. Examples include walking, jogging, jumping rope, bicycling (stationary or outdoor), cross-country skiing, skating, rowing, high- or low-impact aerobics, swimming, and water aerobics.

Healthy Habits

Changes in lifestyle are a crucial component of any blood pressure program. Lifestyle improvements can, in some instances, be the only medication required to reduce blood pressure to acceptable levels.

Changes you want to make when you have high blood pressure include:

- Lose some weight if you are above the healthy weight
- Quit smoking if you are involved in smoking
- Eat a healthy diet rich in low-fat dairy, fruits, and vegetables, and low in saturated fat
- Limit sodium (salt) intake to no more than 2,300 milligrams a day
- Participate in regular aerobic exercise at least thirty minutes a day, most days of the week

- Limit alcohol intake to no more than two drinks a day for men and one drink a day for women

Physical Limitations

Hypertension does not necessarily allow you to limit your activities, to encourage you to engage in the activity, travel, and enjoying life to the maximum.

Many doctors may suggest that you stop unnecessary "thrill rides." And if you have a heart problem that affects your lungs, or if you have trouble breathing, you should avoid things that can shorten your breath.

Emotional

Chronic illnesses of some sort will take an emotional toll over time, whether it's because of the drugs, health screening, changing habits, or something else.

There is a correlation between hypertension and depression, but the link between cause and effect is not well known. If you have depression or a sense of hopelessness for a long time, talk to your doctor. When you are diagnosed with depression, your symptoms can be alleviated by a combination of cognitive therapy, medication, and medical care.

Stress often plays a role in causing hypertension, but from a scientific perspective, the connection is not entirely clear. Whether you have been suffering from chronic stress for years, hypertension can also exacerbate and impede your recovery effort. Stress may be handled by therapy, a change of mind, or medication. Perhaps the best way to deal with stress is to make immediate and practical adjustments in your routine or to change any of your life requirements.

Finally, since hypertension does not cause noticeable symptoms, some people who are affected may fail to take medication or make lifestyle changes that can influence their blood pressure. It is known more frequently by friends and family than by someone who has high blood pressure.

You can seek to speak explicitly about your problems if it sounds like a loved one but be conscious that people are merely responsible for their actions and wellbeing. There is a limit on how much you can get others to decide to take action. If you have hypertension, remember this fact: understanding that denial is a normal and natural diagnostic reaction, but it has to be overcome if you want to live your healthiest life.

Social

Hypertension does not affect one's social life in the way other disorders cause people to miss out on obligations and the like.

However, improvements that can help raise your high blood pressure may have social consequences.

For example, if you have to give up smoking or decrease your consumption of alcohol, it can influence your time with family if your interactions concentrate heavily on those things. Some people with high blood pressure should also not consume many of the foods served at social occasions because they are high in salt, cholesterol, or calories.

This is up to you if you want to explain this to others, but most people with high blood pressure are able to have daily social interactions, possibly with slight changes, rather than restrictions.

Support

Hypertension support groups may be challenging to reach, but you can find some (in person or online) linked to an underlying disorder that triggers hypertension if you have one. Having said that, it is worth asking other people whether they, too, treat high blood pressure if you are open to diagnosis. Many people with high blood pressure share recipes and tips for delicious, blood pressure-lowering dishes, and these experiences are vital as you work towards your objectives.

Practical

You should take some reasonable steps to ensure you meet your treatment targets if you have hypertension. Your blood pressure must be tested (and tracked) periodically, every one to six months, for the efficacy of your medication. You can do so in the doctor's office or probably in a nearby clinic or pharmacy. Some individuals with hypertension find it beneficial to regularly monitor blood pressure with a home blood pressure monitoring system. Generally, these types of tools are straightforward to use and relatively inexpensive. Devices like smartphones, tablets, and smartwatches can save blood pressure records when attached to a blood pressure control system. Most apps can even submit details to your doctor's office or even your health insurance provider (if you choose). Such records will assist your doctor, in particular, if your blood pressure is not steady.

Schedule about Medication

Timing and wear off anti-hypertensive doses can also affect the blood pressure. Generally, the medication should be taken as prescribed, and the dosages should be spaced uniformly over the day if your drugs are regular.

Some people find that taking medicines at specific periods of the day works well for a more extended period to control target blood pressure.

Pay Attention to Blood Pressure Triggers

Some people find that after using salt, their blood pressure rises while others respond to stress or unnecessary physical activity. Know what exactly causes you, and you can do your best, if possible, to prevent these factors.

Conclusion

Hypertension is a common and significant cause of stroke and other cardiovascular disorders. There are many causes of hypertension, such as defined hormonal and genetic syndromes, renal disease, and racial and family factors of multifactorial nature. Blood pressure (BP) is defined as the level of pressure exerted on the artery walls of the blood vessels when the heart contracts against resistance. High BP is regarded as hypertension in a clinical term. Sustained diastolic BP more significant than 90 mmHg or sustained systolic BP greater than 140 mmHg is defined as hypertension. The highest possible arterial strain during contraction of the heart's left ventricle is called systolic BP, and minimal arterial pressure during heart ventricle relaxation and dilation when the blood vessels fill with blood is called diastolic BP. Hypertension is commonly broken down into two secondary and primary hypertension categories. In primary hypertension, sometimes called essential hypertension is defined by chronic blood pressure elevation resulting from another disorder, such as kidney disease, that occurs without elevating Blood pressure. Essential hypertension is a diverse disorder, with different causal factors in different patients leading to high BP. Essential hypertension needs to separate into various syndromes, as the causes of high BP can be recognized in most patients currently diagnosed as having essential hypertension. About 95 percent of patients with hypertension have essential hypertension. While only about 5 to 10 percent of cases of hypertension are believed to result from secondary causes, hypertension is so prevalent that the primary care practitioner is likely to encounter secondary hypertension frequently.

When the blood is pumped via the blood vessels or arteries, these tubal structures exert a force against all the walls. This force, sometimes referred to as blood pressure, can get high, contributing to hypertension, also called high blood pressure. High blood pressure can be due to high intakes of sodium, certain medicines such as over-the-counter cold relief medicines and oral contraceptives, health issues, smoking, obesity, anxiety, sedentary lifestyle, etc. Moreover, hypertension often leads to a higher risk of aneurysm, stroke, heart attack, heart failure, and damage to the kidneys. Patients suffering from untreated high blood pressure cases are at high risk of heart attack and stroke.

Dietary approaches to alter blood pressure should become an essential strategy for promoting cardiovascular health. There is extensive literature proving that blood pressure is affected by multiple independent dietary elements as well as several dietary patterns. The best explanation for lowering blood pressure or preventing high blood pressure through dietary involvement includes implementing a dietary model such as DASH or a Mediterranean diet, consuming less saturated fat and total fat, having more than enough potassium, reducing the amount of sodium in the food, and limiting alcohol use. Other lifestyle factors, such as magnesium and fiber, are likely to affect blood pressure, but the existing evidence to support their recommendation is unfounded. Additional research is warranted that involves population categories and examines the role of many other nutrient factors, right foods, and dietary patterns in hypertension prevention. Despite a dietary pattern's proven benefits, there are many social and cultural forces and corporate interests that affect whether people embrace and adopt such a diet. There is a need for effective clinical and human health measures that integrate changes in individual behaviors that cause sustained changes in diet and environmental conditions that promote and encourage greater access to healthier choices.

References

Health Threats from High Blood Pressure. (2020). Retrieved from https://www.heart.org/en/health-topics/high-blood-pressure/health-threats-from-high-blood-pressure

Hypertensive Heart Disease: Types, Symptoms, and Diagnosis. (2020). Retrieved from https://www.healthline.com/health/hypertensive-heart-disease

Food, T. (2020). Top 10 Natural Foods to Control High Blood Pressure. Retrieved from https://food.ndtv.com/lists/eat-right-cure-high-blood-pressure-724344

Cold, F., Health, E., Disease, H., Disease, L., Management, P., & Conditions, S. et al. (2020). Five Misconceptions about High Blood Pressure. Retrieved from https://www.webmd.com/hypertension-high-blood-pressure/5-misconceptions-about-hypertension#1

Eating with High Blood Pressure. (2020). Retrieved from https://www.healthline.com/health/high-blood-pressure-hypertension/foods-to-avoid#strategies

Cold, F., Health, E., Disease, H., Disease, L., Management, P., & Conditions, S. et al. (2020). Five Misconceptions about High Blood Pressure. Retrieved from https://www.webmd.com/hypertension-high-blood-pressure/5-misconceptions-about-hypertension#1

Hypertensive Crisis: When You Should Call 911 for High Blood Pressure. (2020). Retrieved from https://www.heart.org/en/health-topics/high-blood-pressure/understanding-blood-pressure-readings/hypertensive-crisis-when-you-should-call-911-for-high-blood-pressure

Cold, F., Health, E., Disease, H., Disease, L., Management, P., & Conditions, S. et al. (2020). Lose Weight and Lower Your Blood Pressure. Retrieved from https://www.webmd.com/diet/obesity/features/real-gains-from-losing-weight#2

Weight Loss and Blood Pressure Control (Pro) | Hypertension. (2020). Retrieved from https://www.ahajournals.org/doi/10.1161/HYPERTENSIONAHA.107.094011

Cold, F., Health, E., Disease, H., Disease, L., Management, P., & Conditions, S. et al. (2020). Take Charge of Your Blood Pressure. Retrieved 12 March 2020, from https://www.webmd.com/hypertension-high-blood-pressure/features/take-charge-of-your-blood-pressure#1

Hypertension and Obesity: How Weight-loss affects Hypertension - Obesity Action Coalition. (2020). Retrieved from https://www.obesityaction.org/community/article-library/hypertension-and-obesity-how-weight-loss-affects-hypertension/

Living Well With Hypertension. (2020). Retrieved from https://www.verywellhealth.com/living-well-with-hypertension-1764117

Blood pressure test - Mayo Clinic. (2020). Retrieved from https://www.mayoclinic.org/tests-procedures/blood-pressure-test/about/pac-20393098

Find out how Hypertension differs in Males and Females - iHealth® Official Site for Personal Health Management. (2020). Retrieved from https://ihealthlabs.com/find-hypertension-differs-males-females/

High blood pressure – causes and connection to heart attacks | CardioSecur. (2020). Retrieved from https://www.cardiosecur.com/magazine/specialist-articles-on-the-heart/high-blood-pressure-causes-and-connection-to-heart-attacks